Four-Seasons
Organic Cow Care

Four-Seasons
Organic
Cow Care

Natural Treatments for Year-Round
Herd Health and Productivity

HUBERT J. KARREMAN, V.M.D.

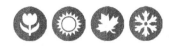

Acres U.S.A.
Austin, Texas

Four-Seasons Organic Cow Care

Copyright © 2016, Hubert J. Karreman, V.M.D.

Acres U.S.A.
P.O. Box 301209
Austin, Texas 78703 U.S.A.
512-892-4400 • fax 512-892-4448
info@acresusa.com • *www.acresusa.com*

Printed in the United States of America

Front cover photography
Tree © dohtar/iStock/Thinkstock
Cow © Can Stock Photo Inc./ VanderWolfImages

CONTENTS

For my daughter

Emily Faith
a gifted writer who has cheerfully proofread
and given clarity to many of the original
writings from which this book was born.
Her wit and humor were evident in her
cartoon drawings along the margins.
With my love and heartfelt thanks.

Preface

For everything there is a season,
and a time for every matter under heaven:
a time to be born, and a time to die;
a time to plant, and a time to pluck up what is planted;
a time to kill, and a time to heal;
a time to break down, and a time to build up;
a time to weep, and a time to laugh;
a time to mourn, and a time to dance;
a time to cast away stones, and a time to gather stones
    together;
a time to embrace, and a time to refrain from embracing;
a time to seek, and a time to lose;
a time to keep, and a time to cast away;
a time to tear, and a time to sew;
a time to keep silence, and a time to speak;
a time to love, and a time to hate;
a time for war, and a time for peace.

Ecclesiastes 3:1–8 (ESV)

This book has taken many years to produce, fifteen to be exact: thirteen years of monthly newsletters and two years of professional editing to combine them in a way that is both timely and educational. I hope the finished product will be enlightening in that you'll be able to immediately utilize this information and work to prevent likely upcoming problems. Certain problems commonly occur at certain times of the year (pasture bloat) while others may happen at any time (hardware)—knowing such things helps in diagnosing an issue. Unfortunately, not all problems can be addressed in any one book, so please keep in mind that these pages only provide a glimpse into the issues that one veterinary practitioner has repeatedly seen affecting organic dairy cows in the northeastern United States.

My publisher, Fred Walters, had the idea that my newsletters ought to be grouped according to seasons—this clicked right away. Fred also came up with the very apt title, *Four-Seasons Organic Cow Care*. This also resonated immediately. Until he had mentioned a working title, I hadn't fully realized how some health care topics do seem to recur with seasonal regularity. Amanda Irle, my editor, merged various similar topics in such a perfect, seamless way that it was actually quite difficult for me to tease apart different years' monthly newsletter entries, except by carefully re-reading each section and realizing how my thinking and use of products had sometimes changed over time.

Many issues visible to the human eye occur on a daily basis, while others we may only detect by the end of a week, and sometimes over a few weeks' time. Some things we never perceive with our eyes, but they happen anyway, like the immune system constantly correcting itself to respond to the unseen and endless challenges we face, whether we are human or animal. With dairy farming being one of the most demanding professions that I know, an entire month or more—indeed "a season"—can pass before certain changes in the farm system, herd, or individual animal are noticed.

Think about the earliest visible signs of spring and how happy that makes us after winter: the reddish color of the swamp maple buds against the dull-gray bark of trees; the tufted mounds of still-dormant grass surrounded by cold saturated soil beginning to appear as the snow recedes; and the swollen, fast-flowing streams reflecting the greening weeping willows along the banks while the nightly frost still leaves frosty blades of grass sparkling in the morning sunlight. Perennial pastures aren't growing yet but wait for the sun to thoroughly warm the earth before emerging from hibernation. Human and animal life again grows more and more active out in the open as warm breezes arrive almost mysteriously . . . and then life finally bursts forth everywhere. All the while, the fragrances of early spring confirm its arrival: the onion-like scent of wild garlic, and the fresh scent of the earth as the ice begins to release its grip on the soil. These are the first impressions of spring, a time when we are more than ready to take in smells other than the warm aroma of the cows in the stable and the old, damp straw bedding piled up nearby.

I happen to write this during a dry spell in August, but as a person who is out and about during all the seasons, I can, in an instant, bring to mind other seasons just by recalling the scents associated with those times. The sense of smell is powerful and connected with our deepest memories—it is a sense that we share with all other animals. By thinking of a specific scent, we can "be there" in that moment once again. Fragrances invoke in us all kinds of emotions. Right now, sycamore trees are releasing their fragrant, cinnamon-like scent into the air, their gigantic leaves the first around here to dry up and turn brown. At first only a single giant leaf rests upon the green carpet of the lawn. More and more leaves join it every day, but still individually scattered, lightly resting upon the grass. When sycamore trees start to change, I am reminded of the beginning of the school year since I walked daily along a street lined with sycamore trees on both sides for ten years, from kindergarten through ninth grade. But it is only during this current time of the season that the sycamores are releasing their aroma to the late summer air. Right now the sun is strong, the ground is dry, and the grass, while still green, is beginning to become slightly brittle. The farmers are getting ready to chop corn silage, barring any unforeseen heavy rains coming from the Southeast or, God forbid, a hurricane that could level a perfect cornfield like those found everywhere around here, with many stalks reaching ten feet tall or more.

It's been a pleasant summer. While the dry May allowed for a lot of really good first-cut traditional dry hay to be made, we had a lot of rain in June to keep the pastures green up to right now in mid-August. It wasn't the hottest of summers here in southeastern Pennsylvania; it was more like what Vermonters would experience as a typical summer. But it was still warm and humid enough for the sudangrass to grow well, even though it wasn't needed as "insurance" against drought (which why it's usually planted). Green native pastures in August *and* sudangrass growing well is an unusually good combination for farmers. I noticed my neighbor getting his third cutting of hay from the small four-acre hayfield behind my house a week ago. He's made dry hay from it once and baleage the other two times. Depending on upcoming weather, the fourth cut will either be the softest hay to feed out during winter or simply be wrapped as ensiled, preserved feed. (If wrapped into a bag and looking like a "marshmallow," its fermented aroma will burst forth when sliced open—yet another fragrance that is easily brought to mind.)

And so it is during the farming seasons: a time to plant and a time to pluck up what is planted; a time to cast away stones and a time to gather stones together; a time to keep and a time to cast away. . . .

While these lines speak to the plant sphere and the seasons I've been describing—either as metaphors or real-life occurrences—they reflect the experience of plant life. But what about the animal sphere? Animals add a complexity to life that plants in their seasonal life and death simply do not. Animals are similar to humans in that they can feel pain and pleasure, sense calm and danger, and instantly react to changes as needed. They move, they chew, they digest, they befriend, they get restless, and they allow humans to handle them. Just by being themselves they affect human well-being. And humans most definitely influence farm animals. The human-animal bond is quite real, whether we are alert and aware of it or numb to it. Humans are usually there when animals come into being and when they pass on: "a time to be born, and a time to die." Indeed, farm animal life is framed and contained by human life. Livestock comes into the world innocently (as all life does) and the whole time it is humans who are in control and ultimately take their life to provide food for others—and during this time humans are completely responsible for their well-being, for their entire life, during health and sickness: "a time to kill and a time to heal." And in a delicate balancing act between species, between those that cannot speak and those that can, we humans need to learn to "listen" in a different way and respond to the best of our ability: "a time to keep silent and a time to speak."

Humans have the capacity to consciously love and can will that love to others, ultimately overcoming internal feelings of hate and arriving at a feeling of true Peace with all life in our midst, whether animal life, plant life or soil or sea life—Creation that God has entrusted to us humans. Indeed, perhaps the greatest mystery of life and the one truly worth all the time and effort to successfully figure out, is finding the source of inner Peace to heal the internal warring which we naturally struggle with as human beings and which too often extends to other Life. Let us not take out our own internal struggles and impatience upon animals—they are innocent of our wrongdoings and simply look to us for their daily needs while returning the favor by providing companionship, milk, fiber, and meat.

At some point in life, I pray that each person begins to feel the keel, rudder, mast, and anchor of God's lifeboat keeping us safe as we navigate through the extremes in life: birth and death, healing and killing, weeping and laughing, mourning and dancing, embracing and refraining from embracing, seeking diligently what is truly needed and becoming willing to lose that which is not needed, dismantling something at one point to learn about it and mending it back together to have it work better, learning how to listen honestly and learning how to speak in kindness (whether by word or by action), overcoming hate with love, and ultimately knowing the Peace that God gives us freely and leaves with us—hoping for us to make the world a better place for all Life that exists, no matter how small or seemingly insignificant.

While the above words may seem lofty to very practical-minded farmers, we become a more whole person when we strive to consciously breathe in life-giving air in a reverent way, noticing slight fragrances and allowing them to mingle with consciousness, emotions, and memory, and then exhaling into the world a part of us that is willing to positively engage with life in our midst, life at all levels—whether soil, mineral, plant, animal or human. We must be open to meeting other life where it is at the moment, without any urge on our part to control or change, simply understanding that life meets us day in and day out, lapsing into weeks and months, beginning and ending seasons that repeat through the cycles of time. How we approach and respond is up to us individually at the heart level. Not surprisingly, it is at the heart level that animals mostly interact, sensing a person's intentions well before the person even sets foot in the pen or walks over to the in-dividual or group. The practical advice held within this book will equip the reader with tools to prepare for the worst so that more time can be devoted to living life to its fullest alongside all the life that calls to us and relies upon us just as we rely on it, life that we will see everywhere if we but stop and deeply breathe in the scent of the seasons.

Introduction

When I decided to no longer write the *Moo News* in January 2013, I had been writing the monthly newsletter for a full thirteen years—about 150 issues in all. The *Moo News* originated as a way for me to give local clients practical tips for health care from what I saw in practice with organic dairy cows. Each issue of the *Moo News* focused on what I was seeing in the field, tips to prevent seasonal problems, and/or what may have been occurring in the organic world generally. In a quick review, I see that I've written a fair number of times on the specific following topics over the years: parasites, flies, grazing, lameness, bloat, various infectious diseases, pinkeye, pneumonia, mastitis, dry cows, obstetrics and uterine problems, calves, digestion and metabolic issues, cow environment, immune system, alternative medicine, research, National Organic Standards Board (NOSB) issues, journeys to different countries, and a few other topics. Many of these articles have made it into this book. I hope readers will learn how to deal with common problems in different ways.

The year 2013 marked my twenty-fifth anniversary of working with organic livestock. Before I had any clue what organic was, I spent four years in college at the University of New Hampshire learning soil science. As a student I had a work-study job at the United States Department of Agriculture (USDA) Soil Conservation Service, now the Natural Resources Conservation Service (NRCS), for two years, helping to survey land and design contour strips, subsurface drainage, farm ponds, woodland access roads, and manure storage facilities in southeastern New Hampshire. While we were surveying, I was fascinated by the cows in the distance. I didn't grow up on a farm, so right after college I apprenticed myself out to farmers for essentially next-to-nothing pay to learn about dairy cows. For four years and a few bucks per hour I mucked out stalls, fixed fences, fed cows with a skid loader, learned to use milking machines, and did other general "hired-hand" work, all prior to any work on an organic farm. I'm always thankful for those experiences, as it let me come into my own way of being with cows.

It was in January 1988 that I attended my first Pennsylvania Farm Show. I found myself talking with somebody who worked at the Chesapeake Bay Foundation. One thing led to another, and I applied and was hired for a new job at the Chester County Conservation District to help survey and install soil conservation structures to help "clean up the bay." As the job start date kept getting pushed back due to funding not coming through from Washington, I thought to myself, "How can I ask farmers to install cost-share conservation measures if it takes so long for money to come in the first place?" I was young and impatient.

Yet again, one thing led to another, and I was very fortunate when someone at my Quaker meetinghouse steered me to Seven Stars Farm, a Demeter-certified biodynamic farm located in Chester County. This position was to be very instrumental on my life's path. Seven Stars was, and still is, a complete system—growing their crops biodynamically (a specialized form of organics) to feed their herd and producing Grade-A yogurt on-farm for natural food stores. I will always consider Seven Stars my "home farm" due to my many formative experiences there.

Almost immediately upon arrival I was introduced to two new concepts: management-intensive grazing and alternative medicines. While I right away liked moving cows to new pasture every twelve hours, I will admit that I had little confidence at first in using the alternative medicines. But I quickly found out how well homeopathic remedies, colostrum-whey products, and botanical infusions and ointments worked—and how you get to know individual cows extremely well in trying to figure out which homeopathics to use. This made me happy since I have always been very much an "animal person." I learned how to give shots (intravenous, intramuscular, and under the skin) and learned artificial insemination, being then able to easily treat uterine infections by infusing colostrum-whey and botanicals. I completely immersed myself in learning natural treatments, and it added a brand new dimension to my life. I wasn't interested in learning how to fix a tractor if it broke, but if a cow broke down I was right there, closely attending to the cow's needs, giving her extra-special attention, and listening carefully to what the local vet would say if he was called in.

Then one day it hit me that the natural therapies were working so well that I wanted to go to vet school to learn "the real thing" and to understand how homeopathy could work. I strongly feel that God gave me this realization, as I still wonder how I ever got accepted into vet school, let alone made it through a grueling four years of extremely difficult work. I became a vet in 1995 and have been focused on working with organic dairy cows ever since.

So that's a brief description of how I got involved with dairy farming. How about you? When did you get interested and involved with farming—conventional or organic? Did you grow up on a farm? Did you shift the way in which you go about farming? Or perhaps, like me, you got interested in agriculture while in school. I must say that my initial entry into agriculture was to simply fulfill one goal: to help feed the world. As I set out to do that, first in college and then by apprenticing myself onto farms, I did start helping to feed the world—and now I do so organically. For not having grown up on a farm, I'm very thankful that my school learning and work experience allowed me to understand both conventional and organic dairy farming.

Regardless of when any of us got our start in agriculture, many changes have occurred to both conventional and organic dairying over the past twenty-five years. In conventional agriculture, it's easy to see that it's become more intensive, with various technologies introduced to help get more and more out of fewer and fewer cows with fewer people involved. Production per cow and income over feed cost are key indicators of a farm's success; the trick is keeping costs low while getting more milk out of the cows. However, cow lifespan has been impacted by the various hidden costs associated with high production and intensive agriculture, and after twenty-five years the Chesapeake Bay still isn't cleaned up—but that's due to more than just agricultural runoff.

In organic agriculture, things have become more "standardized" over the past twenty-five years. When I first heard about the proposed federal rules in 1995, I was happy to hear that there would be a national standard, as individual certifiers with varying attitudes and enforcement made it very difficult for nutritionists, agronomists, and veterinarians to know what was allowed and what was not allowed. While there needed to be some sort of national standard to ensure that customers are getting what they think they are, regulations have unfortunately never gotten away from hair-splitting arguments about material inputs. This is where biodynamics definitely "wins" in that it focuses more on the entire farming system as a living whole— including spiritual aspects—in contrast to examining every little input in excruciating detail as the certified-organic world does. Certifiers *still* can't agree on different inputs, even after the official start of the National Organic Program in 2002. But if you can stay away from the endless debates, organic is a great way to farm and certainly helps to produce food for society in a completely clean way.

Probably the best thing that has occurred in the organic sector within the past twenty-five years is the federal requirement that ruminants must consume, on average, a minimum of 30 percent of their dry matter intake from pasture during the grazing season. This one rule alone will forever separate organic livestock farming from mainstream confinement livestock farming. Grazing simply makes sense for cattle—it's how they are biologically designed to eat and live. The certified organic sector *officially guarantees* this for cattle and other ruminants.

I think the next twenty-five years will see a renewed interest in grazing. The arguments for enhancing omega-3 and conjugated linoleic acid (CLA) levels in milk due to grazing are gaining traction. Moreover, grazing seems to enhance cow lifespan as it provides real exercise, enhanced muscle tone and reduces lameness (compared to keeping cows on concrete). Regardless of farming style, farmers like to have long-lived cows. I hope conventional farmers will at least consider grazing to some degree, if not for cow health then at least for the cheap feed. Of course, it's then an easy step to go organic.

In view of all the changes in dairying over the past twenty-five years as well as whatever may lie ahead, covering the basics will always remain critical. Farmers of any stripe can keep livestock healthier by keeping the animals in direct contact with the land and breathing fresh air, having them graze well-managed pastures whenever possible while feeding high-forage rations during the non-grazing times, and providing dry bedding with appropriate ventilation when animals are housed during the winter. I hope you all take a moment to reflect back and sort out what's worked (and what hasn't), but most importantly try to feel how God's hand has moved in your life and be thankful—even if you sometimes feel removed from feeling His hand—for He is always with you. I hope to see you sometime at an animal health workshop, conference seminar, or pasture walk, somewhere among the cows.

Until then, I hope this book will inform you of the various common problems that tend to crop up in each season. For instance, pasture bloat will be found in the spring most of the time, and heat stroke will be in the summer. Some conditions, such as calving and freshening, though they can happen at any time of year, are placed in the section on spring because many organic/grazing farmers like to take advantage of the lush spring growth to feed the majority of their herd and make the most milk at that time. Other problems, like mastitis, can happen during any season and will be found in the section for All Seasons. With biology and managing animals, there are no hard and fast rules. However, there is a certain rhyme and reason for certain conditions to be associated with certain seasons.

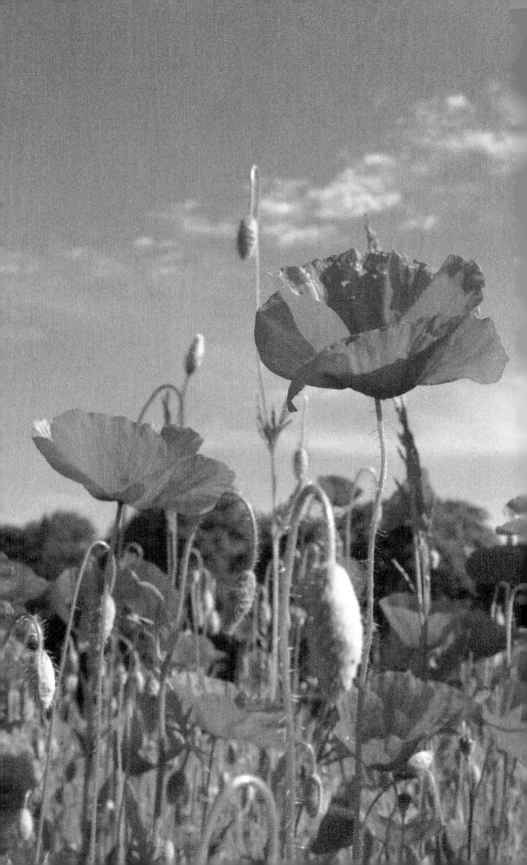

PART I
Spring

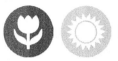

CHAPTER 1

Calving and Freshening

Many farmers tend to have the majority of their cows freshen (give birth) in early spring. This is as it should be, for the pastures will soon be green and lush, providing cows with lots of fresh, alive feed when they need it most—to feed their young. It is interesting to note that the end of pregnancy for most livestock coincides with the beginning of spring. For instance, goats and sheep have a five-month gestation period and are most receptive to becoming pregnant in the autumn, which means lambing/kidding in the spring. Horses have an eleven-month gestation period and are most receptive to becoming pregnant in the spring. Although cows have a nine-month gestation period and can conceive most anytime, just like sows (which have a gestation period just shy of four months), breeding cows in the late spring/early summer (May–June) is usually fairly easy since they are on fresh grass taking in fresh nutrients, which helps the internal hormones associated with fertility to function well. Many farmers take advantage of these naturally occurring phenomena and get the bulk of their herds bred at these times.

Before Freshening

One of the most sensitive times in a cow's life is in the last couple weeks leading up to calving, when the body's natural hormones are rapidly changing in preparation to deliver the newborn. For the dairy farmer, this of course means paying close attention to detail in the last two weeks before freshening, as well as observing proper calving procedures. If all goes well, a cow should calve on her own, drink five to fifteen gallons of water, get up, pass the placenta within four to six hours, start eating, and begin lactation. To have cows hit a decent peak and maintain persistence during lactation, good feeding and body condition is extremely important.

So we should think about the cow's health prior to actually calving. Always have the animal at the farm where she is going to calve for the three weeks prior to actual calving. Do *not* transport her right around calving time. Her immune system isn't very effective at this time to begin with, due to the internal stresses and hormones normally associated with calving, and the strain of transport only makes matters worse. I have seen way too many cows become critically ill when they are bought right at freshening time from a sales stable, and/or they actually calve-in on a cattle hauling truck. At three weeks before calving, we still have time to influence the cow's immune system in a positive way, as indicated by the history of the farm. At this time you want to have the cow where she will be calving so that she will make the correct antibodies for her colostrum.

Colostrum can be positively affected by appropriate use of vaccination, if needed. Any vaccinations that you would like the calf to benefit from can be given to cows two to three weeks before freshening. You may want to vaccinate a cow with a coliform vaccine at this time in order to protect her from getting coliform mastitis when she is just fresh and, secondarily, to enrich the colostrum to protect the calf from deadly coliform scours in its first few weeks of life. If either of these two conditions occurs with some regularity on your farm, seriously consider vaccinating with J-5 or ScourGuard 4KC. If using these two specific products, you must also vaccinate the cow some three to four weeks earlier if it is the first time using it (like a few days prior to drying off). Annual boosters are also effective. For first-calf heifers (whose colostrum is never as enriched with antibodies as a mature cow), consider using a rota/corona vaccine or First Defense, a source of antibodies that can be given orally to newborns if scours in calves always seems to be a problem.

It's also a good time to give MuSe (vitamin E and selenium), which has been scientifically shown to increase immune function, lower somatic cell count when fresh, increase fertility in the coming lactation, and reduce incidence of retained placenta. Retained placentas will unfortunately happen with hard calvings, twins, early calvings, and hypocalcemic (milk fever) cows even if you use MuSe beforehand, but if retained placentas are occurring other than at these times with any regularity, definitely check your selenium levels or simply use an injection of MuSe. These are cheap methods of insurance compared to the costs of lost production and vet bills associated with coliform mastitis treatment or retained placenta/metritis with a possible twisted stomach/displaced abomasum.

One of the biggest factors shown to hinder cows that are coming into third lactation or older is low blood levels of calcium (hypocalcemia/milk fever). This needs to be prevented at all costs as it is a major factor behind a cow not passing the placenta, becoming ketotic, and/or developing a displaced abomasum (twisted stomach). Studies have found that keeping potassium to less than 2.0 percent of the dry cow ration is important in preventing milk fever. Dry cows should not be fed calcium-rich or potassium-rich feeds such as alfalfa. Feeding grassy hay is a great way to accomplish this, but you still need to make sure the hay comes from areas that do not have high potassium in the soil. Grassy hays can indeed have higher amounts of potassium than recommended, especially on farms that have spent lots of money chemical fertilizer over the years in addition to spreading barn manure. In conventional systems, anionic salts are fed to counteract diets high in potassium and calcium; however, they are very unpalatable and need to be "hidden" in the TMR (total mixed ration). Small organic farms might not use TMRs as a feeding strategy and instead use component feeding (feeding each feed sequentially), so the anionic salts aren't able to blend/hide among other feeds. Additionally, anionic salts may not be allowed by some organic certifiers. However, there is a very nice, natural alternative to anionic salts: apple cider vinegar. Feed apple cider vinegar at the rate of two ounces twice daily for two weeks prior to calving (remember the 2-2-2 rule). Apple cider vinegar is acetic acid, which gives off a negatively charged acetate ion, somewhat like the anionic salts. In general, relatively more negative ions (like sulfates) should be fed in during the dry period relative to positive ions (like calcium and potassium), whereas during lactation, relatively more calcium and potassium should be fed compared to the negative ions like sulfates. One interesting ion is magnesium (a positive ion). This should be around 3 percent of the dry cow ration and can be even higher. Magnesium is an incredibly important mineral nutrient for healthy muscles in general, balancing contraction and relaxation in an optimal way.

If severe edema is a problem, you have too many sources of sodium in your dry cow ration (sodium is also a positive ion). Do not give free-choice salt to dry cows, especially not to springing heifers, if udder edema has been an issue on the farm.

Consider teat dipping dry cows within two weeks of freshening twice daily since the keratin plug barriers at the teat ends are softening and environmental bacteria can start to enter the teat canal and cause mastitis. This is especially dangerous during the springtime as the bacteria in the cows' bedding and environment seem to be "waking up" with the warmer temperatures.

Also, springing heifers should start being fed at least some of what the lactating cows are eat-

> **IN GENERAL, RELATIVELY MORE NEGATIVE IONS** (like sulfates) should be fed in during the dry period relative to positive ions (like calcium and potassium), whereas during lactation, relatively more calcium and potassium should be fed compared to the negative ions like sulfates.

ing in terms of hay quality, ensiled feeds, and grain in order to have their rumen bugs adjust. Remember to avoid sudden changes in feed rations at all costs in dairy animals. It takes about two weeks for the rumen bugs to adjust to feed changes.

Okay, that's the pre-game plan. But what about the day-of plan for actual calving?

First of all, try to gauge when a cow will likely freshen. Cows that are within two weeks of freshening need to be observed a few times *daily* for loosening of the ligaments near the vulva as well as general feed intake, especially in bull-bred herds when the exact breeding dates are not known. Additionally, cows diagnosed as possibly having twins should be watched especially carefully as they tend to calve one to two weeks earlier than the expected due date. Cows that are getting ready to calve will begin to eat less at about twelve hours prior to calving. The vulva will look somewhat fuller and looser as well. Milk may be dripping from the teats for a few days beforehand (*definitely* dip teats if dripping). Normal signs also include gradual "bagging-up" over a couple weeks' time (udder enlarges) and a softening of the ligaments between the tail and pin bones.

Some older cows bag up real quickly right before calving. Beware: these older cows likely become milk fever cases. I've seen it often. This occurs because all of a sudden at calving the bones are called upon to release lots of calcium into the bloodstream, and they are simply not able to do so at the rate needed. Then the bloodstream calcium levels become very low and the older cow either gets a slow start or goes down with real milk fever. It is much better to see a cow "bag up" over a few weeks time because to give her bones time to adjust to releasing increasing amounts of calcium into the bloodstream instead of an instant demand right at calving time. Severe amounts of fluid accumulation in front of and in the udder in springing heifers are usually due to free-choice salt: getting too much and then drinking a lot of water and retaining it (due to the salt in the system). In these cases the suspensory ligament of the udder may rupture and the udder will forever be damaged. It may be good to use an udder bra/support on these animals (any lactation or age).

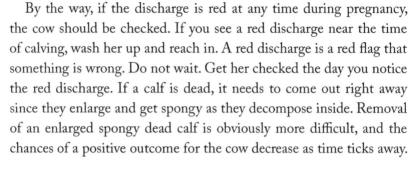

By the way, if the discharge is red at any time during pregnancy, the cow should be checked. If you see a red discharge near the time of calving, wash her up and reach in. A red discharge is a red flag that something is wrong. Do not wait. Get her checked the day you notice the red discharge. If a calf is dead, it needs to come out right away since they enlarge and get spongy as they decompose inside. Removal of an enlarged spongy dead calf is obviously more difficult, and the chances of a positive outcome for the cow decrease as time ticks away.

Calving Area

Cows should be allowed to separate themselves from the group when calving is obviously imminent. If you see a cow that is just beginning to show signs of calving, do not move her to some other area if you can avoid it. Doing so can delay calving twelve hours (resulting possibly in a dead calf being born) as the cow will stop the calving process to reorient herself to her new surroundings.

I know some folks will have more than one cow a day freshening, but that is no excuse not to provide a clean area for calving. Calving outdoors on clean, green grass is ideal, weather permitting. An indoor calving area must at least be dry with a lot of new straw or fodder. Box stalls are not ideal, but also not impossible. When cleaning out the box stall between calvings, lay down a thick coating of lime (Barn-Dri or Barn-Grip) to alter the ground pH and fatally upset the bacterial habitat. I realize that not all box stalls get cleaned out between calvings (although they should!), but spongy bedding is a recipe for health disasters in both cow and calf. The best kind of bedding is straw or fodder. Sand is ideal, but it's not available in all areas. Chopped paper sticks to everything that is wet, and sawdust can harbor coliform bugs that can enter a leaking teat when the cow is lying down. Calving in filth is not smart. Wet, mucky filth coming in contact with a dripping udder spells trouble for the cow as well as likely disease for the newborn calf (navel infection and/or intestinal diseases like coliform, salmonella, and Johne's). If possible, dip the calf's navel in iodine a couple times a day for the first few days (just like a baby), so it quickly dries up nice and crisp. I realize the cow may lick it off, but its antiseptic action upon contact far outweighs the potential health problems that crop up from navel infections (i.e., joint ill giving a swollen joint or joints) that are near impossible to clear up. Lay down lime and bed well between cows that are calving. Of course fresh green pasture is great—but there won't be any in early spring! It is either frozen or mud. Harsh, winter winds or raw, chilly air will diminish a newborn calf's chance to thrive. Calf jackets are great for any wet/damp calf born outside that is weak.

I realize that many of these instructions are easier said than done, but in early spring the weather and ground can be very cold and damp, so consideration must be given to what is in the best interest of both cow and calf if you are making your living as a dairy farmer. Remember that calving time is the most stressful for the cow and is obviously of critical importance to the start of the newborn calf.

Delivery

Okay, so you have the cow and the area prepared. Watch for the cow to eat less about twelve hours before calving; she may lay down more but also quickly get back up, her udder may drip milk (it may for a few days sometimes), and things will greatly loosen up around the tail head. After the water bag breaks, pushing out the calf normally takes about one to three hours but can last up to eight hours (probably in a first-calf heifer or a low-calcium older cow). The mucus should be straw-colored, clear, and thick. If you are not certain how things are progressing, by all means reach in! Get a halter on her, tie her to a post or gate, wash up the vulva well, put on an OB sleeve, lube your arm, and *carefully* reach in (if at any time she passes manure prior to inserting your arm, wash her up again). You should be especially attentive if a cow has her tail out and you can see her pushing but not progressing over a few hours time. This almost always means something is wrong. Another sign that something is wrong is when a red discharge is seen from the vulva and it is not near her calving date, or, when she has a red discharge and is pushing but not progressing.

Okay, so you now have your hand and arm in the cow's birth canal. What do you feel? Is the cervix fully open/dilated or is there a constriction? If the cervix is fully open and you can easily slide your hand into the uterus itself, what do you then notice about the calf? Normal presentations for a calf are either frontward with the head and both front hooves coming towards you or backward with both back hooves coming towards you. Any other position needs correcting prior to extracting the calf.

So, if you feel two hooves and the head—great, allow the calving to proceed. Don't rush a normal, frontward calving, *especially* not with a first-calf heifer. You must allow the birth canal/vagina to expand to accommodate the calf which must pass through it. An animal calving for the first time needs to have the calf's head be in the birth canal long enough to dilate the birth canal effectively; otherwise rips can occur, which can be fatal if they extend to deeply into the tissue surrounding the birth canal or too far forward beyond the cervical-uterine junction. Though not commonly fatal, those rips and tears can really make for a very slow start for her lactation. If you add in corn silage and grain and keep her tied in her stall without normal walking about (exercise), you will have quickly created prime conditions for a twisted stomach/displaced abomasum.

Obviously a live calf is great, but getting one pulled out as fast as possible from a first-calf heifer may lead to the demise of the young cow. Think of it this way: you have invested a lot of money over two years to raise that springing heifer to freshen. You can either ruin her in one quick moment of impatience, or you may lose the calf but have a healthy milking heifer. Have patience!

Problems during Calving

Do you feel only two hooves when reaching in? If the bottom of the hooves are facing down, you are probably feeling the front ones; the bottoms of back hooves usually face upwards towards the sky. If you feel front legs and no head, don't pull without first knowing where the head is. Never, ever pull out a frontwards facing calf without knowing and/or guiding the head to come straight out along with the legs. Always, always, always make sure the head is coming through the cervix while pulling on the legs. I rely quite often on my head snare/loop to make sure the head isn't turning back. If the head is still in the uterus and the legs are being pulled, the head often will turn if the nose is not directed into the cervical tunnel. This is especially true if the calf is dead already.

If you feel the tail with the two hooves, the calf is backward and you can go ahead and pull. Backwards calves are technically normal except that the umbilical cord tends to snap earlier while the calf's head is still in the uterus, which leads to the calf drowning in the uterine fluids. If you only feel the tail, it is a breech birth and needs veterinary attention. A cow will never be able to calve-in a breech birth on her own, *never*. If you feel one leg "turned back" (with the hoof going towards the cow's head, carefully cup your hand over the hoof and bend the leg the way it naturally wants to bend. Bring the hoof close in towards the calf's belly and then bring the hoof toward you. *Always* cup the hoof in the palm of your hand to avoid unnecessary rips to the uterus. A rip in the uterus is generally fatal, even with antibiotics. *Always* have the cow standing (if you can) when you go to rearrange limbs—it is much easier to rearrange limbs with the cow standing. If the cow is lying down, the floor is blocking a potential area of movement. Standing up while working on a standing cow is also nicer than kneeling in damp bedding.

It is not too difficult to rearrange a leg that is turned back, but you have to reach in the cow first to find the problem. If you do not reach in, you will not know what is happening and be unable to make a rational decision about the situation at hand. Never hesitate to call a veterinarian when it comes to calving questions. I have helped many farmers with calving questions over the phone when they call and describe what they are feeling inside the cow. While not always successful in helping them out over the phone, it has reduced some driving out to farms late at night, much to the appreciation of the farmer.

Once the calf's head and front legs are out of the cow to the "armpits" of the calf, stop everything for a moment. Cross the front legs of the calf and turn the calf slightly so that it will be delivered with its backbone eleven o'clock or one o'clock to the cow's backbone. Doing this is incredibly important in preventing hip lock. Hip lock is when the calf's hips become stuck during calving and only a very forceful extraction can free it up to come fully out. Cross the front legs of a few calves being born for a few calvings and you'll agree that the calvings go easier. The pelvic outlet is shaped like an upside-down egg, and the calf's hook bones will pass out much easier if the calf is slightly turned. It will save many a cow from a pinched nerve and being down, especially first-calf heifers which are naturally smaller animals than more mature cows.

Once delivered, take the calf by the back legs and swing it around 360 degrees a few times (until you get dizzy). Or lay the calf on the cow's back with the calf's nose low to the ground. These two methods allow any fluids that it might have sucked in while still inside the cow to drain out of the calf's windpipe or throat.

Always check for a twin, especially if the calf is somewhat small or the cow is early by a week or two.

After you give the cow five to ten gallons of lukewarm water, which a normal cow will suck right down, get the cow to stand up. This is to check to see if she can indeed stand up (as she should be able to) and can help prevent a prolapsed uterus as the uterus will hang down inside the belly better when she is standing rather than possibly flopping out of a lying down cow—especially if her rump is facing downhill.

If a cow looks like she is straining to calf and is not advancing at all for about two to three hours, she may have a twisted uterus/ uterine torsion. Uterine torsions are extremely common—especially in the Holstein breed. There might be trouble if you notice that the cow has its tail out, not resting upon itself like normal, and the cow shows some pushing but no progress. Wash her up and reach in with an OB sleeve and lube. If you feel a turning or auger-like feeling as you reach through the cervix for the calf, there is a good chance there is a torsion present. By carefully feeling with your finger tips along the floor and walls of the birth canal and into the cervix, you will notice a turning, corkscrew-like effect as the birth canal tightens down. Usually farmers will say that the calf feels like it is really "far in" before they can reach it. Call for assistance as a cow will *never* be able to calve on her own with a twisted uterus. The longer you wait, the lower your chance of having a live calf. Do not wait and see. Live calves are a very common ending to a corrected uterine torsion. If the calf is alive prior to correction of the uterine torsion, it will likely be born alive once the torsion is corrected. If it is already dead before correcting the uterine torsion, it will need to be extracted right after the correction as the cervix will start to close down.

If you reach in the first moment you suspect a problem and call for help in time there will be a better outcome. Correcting a uterine torsion is actually kind of fun for me as a veterinarian. There are a few ways to correct a uterine torsion, and all are very manual. The first step is to determine which direction the torsion is going. You don't need to know "left or right" or "clockwise or counterclockwise"; simply reach your hand and arm inside the birth canal and literally feel which way the auger-like corkscrew turning is going. Once you do, you will need to "cast the cow" down onto the ground and roll her *the direction the twist is going* (the direction you felt when reaching in her). Roll her over her back in that direction. You will need two people minimum—one person rolling her front half and the second person rolling her back legs (be careful, but they often give up once being rolled). It is ideal to have a third person, usually the veterinarian, sit on the cow's belly just in front of

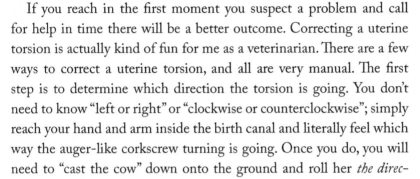

ONCE DELIVERED, take the calf by the back legs and swing it around 360 degrees a few times (until you get dizzy).

the udder to keep the calf in place while the cow is rolled to correct the torsion. Once rolled, stand the cow back up, clean her vulva up as needed and reach in. Often times, with just one roll, the auger-like feel will be gone and there is a direct open path for the calf to come out. Sometimes the rolling needs to be done a few times. It is important to stand the cow up after each roll and reach in to check if the torsion has been corrected. If only two people are rolling the cow, the rolling itself should be done in a quick motion for the best results. Granted, my preferred method is when I can flip the calf over with my forearm inside the uterus of a standing cow and thereby correct the torsion. But this takes some practice at becoming proficient, whereas rolling a cow is a tried and true method.

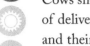

Cleaning

Cows should pass the entire placenta ("clean") within four to six hours of delivery. Cows will do this if there is a normal unassisted delivery and their blood calcium levels are normal. If a cow that hasn't passed her placenta in the normal six hours, put her calf (or another calf) with her and let the calf suck on the cow's udder as often as it wants. This will generally help the uterus contract and push out the placenta. If a placenta sits in the uterus too long, sometimes for days on end, it will putrefy and cause many complications to the just-fresh cow. Many people and animals have died over the millennia due to uterine infections. Dairy farmers who raise calves on cows often observe that there aren't retained placenta problems anymore. I'm not certain how often beef cattle have retained placentas, but I doubt it occurs as frequently because beef calves are allowed to suck on their moms freely (causing oxytocin contractions of the uterus).

Even if a cow totally expels the placenta on the second or third day fresh, she usually ends up having a uterine infection. Uterine infections need to be treated promptly and effectively within the first

The Reproductive Cow Clock

The Reproductive Cow Clock is a simplified version of the actual reproductive cycle of a bovine. Anatomically, the female reproductive tract begins with the ovaries, of which there are two (left and right). These are connected to the uterus by way of the oviduct. The uterus also has a right and left side (better known as "horns" due to their general shape). Then there is the main body of the uterus, which is sealed off from the outside world by the cervix. Only when in heat or when giving birth should the cervix allow the uterus and the outer world to be directly connected. The birth canal (vagina) is on the opposite side of the cervix from the uterus, and then there is the vulva, which is visible from behind the cow. The cow's urethra enters the floor of the vagina to allow the cow to urinate. When

Cow Clock (± 21 days)

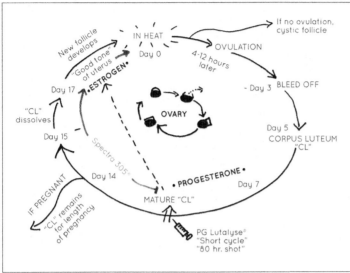
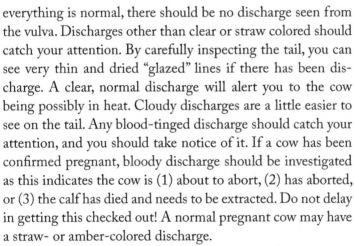

everything is normal, there should be no discharge seen from the vulva. Discharges other than clear or straw colored should catch your attention. By carefully inspecting the tail, you can see very thin and dried "glazed" lines if there has been discharge. A clear, normal discharge will alert you to the cow being possibly in heat. Cloudy discharges are a little easier to see on the tail. Any blood-tinged discharge should catch your attention, and you should take notice of it. If a cow has been confirmed pregnant, bloody discharge should be investigated as this indicates the cow is (1) about to abort, (2) has aborted, or (3) the calf has died and needs to be extracted. Do not delay in getting this checked out! A normal pregnant cow may have a straw- or amber-colored discharge.

As for the reproductive cycle itself, there will be a dominant follicle that contains the egg to be fertilized during the current estrus (heat) cycle. There are other small follicles that can "present themselves" within the twenty-one-day cycle, and any one of those small follicles can give slight "tone" to the uterus, faking out a vet as to predicting when a cow will actually come in heat. The presence of the CL (corpus luteum) suppresses these small follicular waves until the CL itself dissolves around day seventeen if not pregnant (or is eliminated by a short cycle injection of PGF2$_\alpha$). Cysts will interfere with the normal clock and must be treated, either by being gently ruptured manually by a veterinarian, given a natural treatment like homeopathic Apis (if a right-sided cyst) or lachesis (if a left-sided cyst), acupuncture, or eliminated by an injection of gonadorelin-releasing hormone (GnRH). Both the injections mentioned are prohibited for use in the U.S. organic livestock sector but allowed with restrictions in Canada and the EU organic livestock sector. Cows that are skinny simply will not cycle in general until the likely negative energy balance is corrected. There are no treatments except to get more condition on the cow.

fourteen days fresh in order to avoid a long-standing uterine infection going into lactation. U.S. organic farms must be particularly vigilant because the typical hormonal therapy prostaglandin F2$_\alpha$ (Lutalyse) is prohibited in the United States (it is not prohibited for therapeutic use in Canada and the European Union). Conventional farms are lucky that they can use PG/Lutalyse therapeutically at day fourteen fresh to help "clean up" a uterus, which is what PGF2$_\alpha$ (prostaglandin) was originally discovered to do. Prior to that, the only way cows could be effectively treated for a bad uterus would be with antibiotic infusions. This is simply not a first-choice option on organic farms in the United States (although it could be used in the European Union). If antibiotics are used on an organic dairy cow in Canada, then there is a thirty-day milk withholding time.

If an older cow (third lactation or older) has a normal, unassisted delivery and does not clean, strongly consider giving calcium. Calcium levels not only affect the leg muscles (thus the cow's ability to properly rise), they also affect all muscles: uterine muscles (to expel calf and cleanings), muscles surrounding the rumen and abomasum (to help proper digestion), muscles that control the teat sphincters (to help keep teats from leaking), as well as the muscles that constrict or dilate the pupil. Low-calcium cows will have dilated pupils, trembling/twitching skin near the shoulders or thighs, be a little dull, not clean, and perhaps mildly bloated; they can be low in calcium even though they are standing up and eating a little.

It is absolutely critical to treat the cow's uterus with antiseptics (like iodine)—make sure you do it and repeat it daily. The cervix is usually open enough to pass your antiseptic through into the uterus until about the tenth to fourteenth day fresh. A hand can usually pass directly into the uterus until about day five after calving, and after that pills or infusion rods can still be passed carefully through the cervix. If a cow has an infected uterus, she should be treated *at least* three to four different days prior to day ten fresh and ideally every single day that it's possible to place a treatment into the uterine environment.

Unfortunately, I have seen organic cows leave the herd due to long-standing uterine infections that could have been prevented if effectively treated during the first two weeks of lactation. Most cows that are found to have an infected uterus at three to four months into lactation are very difficult to effectively treat. While there may be a cow or two that has gotten over a bad uterus with treatment only started far into lactation, most others are not so lucky—and I have tried a variety of approaches. Other veterinarians working with organic herds have, too, but to no avail. When I feel a uterus full of pus at four to six months into lactation, I am always saddened to hear that the cow was treated only one time right after calving, even though the farmer knew she had a bad uterus at that time. A retained placenta and ensuing uterine infection is probably the only time in natural farming systems when a timely and true action has to be taken in order to avert an entirely preventable and ultimately intractable chronic condition. By making sure that calcium levels are adequate, calving areas (and potential procedures) are clean and hygienic, and that we jump on uterine problems early and often, reproductive fertility on organic farms can be easily maintained.

Conclusion

Bovine obstetrics is an art. There is no exact science to it. A little care, patience, and compassion will go a long way. If you feel uncomfortable about a certain situation, don't hesitate to call your vet, as I for one find obstetrics cases some of the most interesting. I like to help calve-in problem cows that I called pregnant. It seems only right to follow through for all phases of a cow's life. Delivering a live calf while protecting the cow is obviously the goal, but while it is not always possible to get a live calf, compassionate care for the cow is paramount and my highest concern. It should be the farmer's as well.

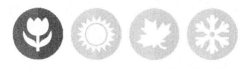

CHAPTER 2

Calf Care

There are lots and lots of calves born in the spring, and with good reason—there is a fresh supply of food from to keep mom healthy and feeding her calf. Of course, that's the general biology of many species, not only cows. While the last chapter concentrated on the cows and their difficulties at calving time, here we will discuss the newborn calves and overcoming challenges they may face.

Environment

The number one cardinal rule to remember with calves: clean and dry bedding with good ventilation. Actually that goes for all animals, but especially young stock. In general, hutches are a great way to reduce disease in calves (if not nursing on cows). Penned calves within the barn are the most likely to come down with typical problems like scours and pneumonia. Have calves outside in fresh air as soon as possible. Pneumonia is a real threat, especially in the changing season when damp, chilly air just around freezing is likely.

Let's talk about calves on pasture. First, always try to have calves on "clean pasture," meaning that adult cows haven't been on it for a couple years, and neither have other calves. This is very difficult to do in practice. Therefore, at minimum do *not* follow adult cows immediately with younger animals; this not only increases parasite pressure on the young stock but also increases the likelihood of Johne's transmission to the young stock, if Johne's is a problem in the herd. While people know that some internal parasites can overwinter in the soil, not many people know that the Johne's bacteria can also remain viable in the soil for more than a year. Many people will clip pastures in order to splatter out manure pies so the parasites and other germs dry up in the sun and wind (as well as to give a uniform regrowth of the paddock). If you do not like to clip pasture, then I suggest that you have poultry to peck and scratch at the manure pies. Hogs will also gladly root through manure pies in search of grain and/or minerals. You could also follow with other ruminants, as most internal parasites are species specific, but that will not destroy the existing cow pies like clipping or having poultry or hogs work on them would.

Also, once calves are put outside (individual hutches, group hutches, or with cows) do *not* bring them back inside until they're ready to freshen. Why? Stale barn air is very difficult on an animal's system, especially if they have internal parasites. The intranasal vaccines (TSV-2, Nasalgen, and InForce 3) are all excellent at preventing respiratory disease/shipping fever and should be given about three to four days prior to mixing animals and/or placing animals in conditions without fresh air.

Feeding and Nutrition

Make sure newborn calves are getting a gallon of colostrum in them within the first six to eight hours of life. This is not impossible, and it is your responsibility to make sure it happens! You *must* take advantage of the open and accepting gut during this critical time. If the calf does not suck for whatever reason, use a commercial calf tube feeder to get the needed colostrum into it. Don't freely pour it into the calf's mouth—that is a sure recipe for getting it into the windpipe. If you are not sure whether the calf got colostrum, don't hesitate to give it a bottle or tube feed it. When tube feeding a calf (remember that when straddling the calf with the head in front of you, your left is its left), pass the tube *left of center* into the mouth and into its throat. There is no substitute for the required amount of colostrum. In general, the oldest cows will have the richest colostrum.

If the cow died during birth and there are no other fresh cows with colostrum, use a commercial source of antibodies (First Defense capsules) as soon as possible (not tomorrow, it will be too late!).

The calf's gut is very receptive to the large antibody molecules in colostrum and is porous enough to allow them to be absorbed intact into the bloodstream from the intestine—but *only* in the first twenty-four to thirty-six hours after birth. Unfortunately, disease-causing germs (E. coli, rotacorona virus, salmonella, Johne's, etc.) can also pass through the calf's intestinal wall at this time, so it is absolutely critical that you have cows calve in clean and dry surroundings.

The best way to prevent baby calf problems is to run them at their mom's side or with other nurse cows, and preferably outside. If that's not possible or desirable, keeping a calf with its mom for a week will at least allow for a healthy bonding to occur, yet not so much so as when keeping a calf with a cow until weaning. Keeping a calf with its mom allows vigorous nursing many times a day—good for both calf and mom. Why? The calf will take in many small, frequent meals instead of just being fed a large slug twice daily, which can cause digestive upset. Multiple meals will also satisfy the calf's urge to suck and therefore reduce its urge to potentially suck on pen mates. The cow will release natural oxytocin in response to the calf as it bumps up to the udder to suck, which will help a first-calf heifer learn to let her milk down. Perhaps more importantly, the oxytocin release will help the uterus contract and shrink down to normal size more quickly. Therefore, if you have a first-calf

> **THE CALF'S GUT IS VERY RECEPTIVE** to the large antibody molecules in colostrum and is porous enough to allow them to be absorbed intact into the bloodstream from the intestine—but only in the first twenty-four to thirty-six hours after birth.

heifer that won't let her milk down, put a calf on her and it should help. If this is not possible, vigorously stimulate the cow's teats and udder, even bumping up against it with your fist, just as a calf does when it is searching for the teat (like those calves that bump up against you whenever they get a chance). That kind of physical interaction will give the brain a stronger signal to release oxytocin than just quickly washing the four teats and stripping out a few shots of milk. Another way to get a cow to let her milk down, especially a first-calf heifer, is to put a sleeve on and reach in rectally, like a veterinarian does for a pregnancy check. Running your arm in and out over the cervix area a few times will trigger the cervix to send a signal to the brain to let milk down. This is basically mimicking what happens when a calf is about to be born and bumps up against the cervix from the inside: the cow starts to drip milk for the calf (even though it's not quite there yet to suck on the udder).

Calves tend to be the healthiest when on nurse cows. This is not rocket science; it's what Mother Nature intended. These calves are generally the strongest, healthiest, and fastest growing of any I've ever seen. There are a few things to keep in mind when selecting appropriate nurse cows. First, they should be negative for Johne's disease, which is easily transmitted in milk directly from the udder. Cows that are high in somatic cell count but don't have outright mastitis and those cows that have lopsided udders or are three-teated are potential nurse cows as well. Some farmers are adamant about only using nurse cows with the highest-quality milk for calves, and this is certainly understandable, but using nurse cows with lower-quality milk will still produce a very healthy and vigorous calf.

When running calves with cows, use fresh cows and start with three calves per cow, but at about a month into it, drop back to two calves per cow, as they do drink a lot. You still need to feed these nurse cows well as they must make milk for the calves and are being drained out continuously. Perhaps a good trial would be to keep a few calves with their moms for the first week; I would guess that the calves will get out of the starting gate wonderfully and incidences of retained placenta will drop to near zero. Perhaps you'll decide to try a small group of nurse cows and calves and see how it goes—I predict that those calves will be pictures of health.

If using bottles and nipples, make sure that the bottles and mob feeder are clean. The germs found in dirty bottles and mob feeders would amaze you. The excuse that you've gotten away with not cleaning them for long stretches in the past does not hold up if there are problems occurring right here and now. Action must be taken or you will simply keep adding to the germ load. Don't think of it as a hassle to keep these items clean. Calves are very sensitive to their environment, lack a competent immune system, and are totally dependent on our good care. They are your future herd.

Calf Nutrition Q&A

If you still have questions about calf nutrition, review and consider the following suggestions:

Q: The cow died during calving (or has no milk), and the calf didn't get colostrum. What can I do?

A: Use colostrum from another cow (preferably an older one) or use a First Defense bolus (commercial source of antibodies) within the first six to twelve hours of life.

Q: Who is feeding the calf?

A: You are, not the children, especially if there are problems.

Q: When is the calf being fed?

A: At the same times, always. Do not vary.

Q: What is the calf being fed?

A: Whole milk. Also offer hay from day one. The calf's immature rumen absolutely must have fibrous stems and roughage for it to develop and become functional as quickly as possible. Consider baby beef calves with their moms on pasture—they are already chewing cud at one to two weeks of age as well as learning grazing behavior that will last a lifetime. Simply put, calves with a functional rumen can withstand many more of life's stresses (especially gut challenges) than those only getting milk replacer and grain. I will stick my neck out here and say that those nutritionists who advocate withholding hay from calves until they are a month old have no clue as to the developmental biol-

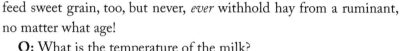

ogy of calves. Ever see calves nibbling their bedding? That is the behavior of calves desperately seeking to satisfy an intense natural craving for fiber. They know they need it. Case closed. Of course you may feed sweet grain, too, but never, *ever* withhold hay from a ruminant, no matter what age!

Q: What is the temperature of the milk?

A: Body temp (102°F) every single time, not cold.

Q: What height are they being fed milk?

A: About nose height, right like a calf would suck from a cow's udder, never ground level.

If you are still experiencing problems, do not wait until the calf is flat out and severely dehydrated. Act at the first sign that they are not vigorously drinking. Calves have little to no reserves. Prompt attention and action on your part is required. Waiting twelve to twenty-four hours to see if they "come around" is an especially not bright idea regarding calves since they have so few body reserves.

If you see white scours and they are one to fourteen days old, the cause is usually E.coli bacteria or rota-coronavirus. They both can kill, but E.coli does it more quickly due to the bacteremia (blood poisoning). You can get a calf over rota-coronavirus by paying strict attention to the hydration of the calf—learning to tube feed a calf is thus an essential part of calf husbandry. I've already described the practice earlier in this chapter, but rest assured that tube feeding a calf is not rocket science. Animals with E.coli need the same care as rota-corona animals but also antibodies to E.coli (multi-serum, Bovi-Sera).

Calf Problems

February through March is a big time for calving but, depending on your location, a terrible time for calves to be born, in a sense. Although God intended herbivores (cows, horses, sheep, goats) to give birth in the spring, He meant it to coincide with abundant, nutritious feed in the form of pasture, which isn't the case every year. Calves can too easily become damp and chilly, which weakens them immensely. April, although often pleasant during the day in southeastern Pennsylvania, can certainly be rainy and cold as well, especially at night. At the first sign of a calf not finishing its bottle or not staying at the mob feeder, take its temperature, check its rear end and back legs for typical scours/wetness, and pinch its eyebrow to assess its hydration. Its hydration is okay if the eyebrow does not stay pinched up after you are done pinching and let go—the longer it stays pinched up, the worse the dehydration. Also check the rate of breathing. If there are no obvious signs of scours, the problem is probably pneumonia, but they can have both at the same time (a very bad situation).

If a calf does get scours within the first twelve days of life, it is almost always due to rota-coronavirus or E.coli bacteria. The first thing to do is to feed calves fluids more often than the routine twice a day, since they will definitely have bouts of diarrhea more than twice a day. Give about two-thirds the volume of a normal feeding, but feed four times a day, alternating between milk and electrolytes each time.

A quick and handy homemade electrolyte mix consists of one gallon of water, two teaspoons baking soda, two teaspoons salt, and eight tablespoons honey.

If the calf is too weak to suck the bottle, you must tube feed it or it will wither quickly.

If calves typically get scours by a certain day of life on your farm, try vaccinating the dry cows as discussed in chapter 6, and/or give the proven immune stimulant ImmunoBoost 1cc under the skin a day or two prior to "usual" outbreak time. If scours is still a problem, give a treatment dose of about 50–75cc Bovi-Sera or multi-serum—both sources of antibodies against typical scours and pneumonia-causing bugs that cattle of any age commonly encounter. You should repeat the next day; these antibodies will slowly decline over seven to ten days. Better yet is to give both the first and second day doses together at once the first day. This is to get the highest level of antibodies right in the beginning of therapy.

Fluid therapy is critical to any young calf with scours, no matter what bacteria or virus causing it. You either do it orally or you'll need the vet to give IV fluids, which usually is usually a combination of 800cc lactated ringers solution, 100cc dextrose, and 100cc sodium bicarb.

Scours due to parasites include the protozoal coccidia, cryptosporidia, and giardia types and the nematode/helminth stomach worms. Affected calves usually display an enlarged belly, rough hair, manure splattered and dried on their back legs, and occasionally coughing. The scours is usually dark with red streaks in coccidia, and the calf strains. Parasitic infestations are commonly seen just after the stress of weaning, but it certainly can occur earlier. Pens of calves kept within the main barn or batches of calves continually using the same exact location invite parasite infections. In group pens, try to sanitize the area before new calves occupy it. In hutches, move them to new locations, use some gravel to help ground drainage, and turn up unused hutches to get the benefit of the sun's ultraviolet rays to sanitize. Manure samples should be analyzed to diagnose the parasite. Most dairy vets do this right at the office. Coccidiostats like amprolium work well for coccidia. These aren't allowed on organic farms, so I try a product called Ferro, an "earth tea" which is extremely high in iron and scores of other minerals. This stops the diarrhea and also replenishes iron to the little calf's system in a biologically friendly way. Ferro is beneficial in stomach worm problems. Although it doesn't necessarily kill worms, it makes the intestinal terrain inhospitable through gut spasm, and it seems as though they release their "grip" on the gut. It also replenishes iron to the system, which becomes severely anemic due to worm infestations. Of course, regular wormers work as well, but there is evidence of growing resistance to them. Organic farmers are allowed to use ivermectin, moxidectin, or fenbendazole in an emergency when methods acceptable to organic have failed. Sometimes if you use ivermectin, moxidectin, or fenbendazole to worm a calf suffering from both stomach worms and coccidia, the calf will be less stressed once the stomach worms are killed and can then overcome the coccidia with its own immune

A QUICK AND HANDY HOMEMADE ELECTROLYTE MIX consists of one gallon of water, two teaspoons baking soda, two teaspoons salt, and eight tablespoons honey.

system. It is when they are parasitized with both coccidia and worms that they become overwhelmed. See the chapter on parasitism for more information.

Calf Scours Q & A

If you are still experiencing problems with calf scours, review and consider the following suggestions:

Q: Which calves are getting sick? The ones from first-calf heifers?

A: If yes, then consider vaccinating the springing heifers three weeks before calving with ScourGuard 4KC or J-5 to boost the antibody content of the colostrum.

Q: Don't feel like catching up springing heifers to vaccinate them?

A: You really need to.

Q: What should I feed a calf with scours?

A: Electrolytes only, no milk for twenty-four to thirty-six hours, then slowly add back in real, whole milk. Feed electrolytes, half a bottle four times a day, then the same amount and frequency when adding back in whole milk. The electrolytes can be as simple as the honey and baking soda recipe given earlier in this chapter.

Conclusion

It is with calves raised as Mother Nature would that it's truly easiest to see robust health. Put some calves on cows this coming season and observe this for yourself.

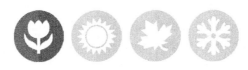

CHAPTER 3

Ketosis and the Energy Needs of Lactating Cows

As we get into grazing time, I want to talk a little about the energy needs of lactating cows. As we all know, the protein content of fresh, growing pasture plants is high. Protein contains nitrogen. If lots of protein/nitrogen are going into the rumen, you need to have a corresponding amount of energy/carbon (=carbohydrate) to balance it out. Just like the soil and its microbes need a certain carbon-to-nitrogen ratio to be in optimal balance, so, too, does the rumen and its microbes. Part of the breakdown of soluble protein in the rumen creates urea, which is eventually converted to urine and then excreted. This is not a "free" process; there's always a biological cost to the cow processing protein nitrogen in terms of energy for metabolism, which can deplete the cow and leave it very skinny and producing lots of loose manure. There is no way to keep up with actual milk production in these circumstances since energy is also needed in a big way for milk production.

Two things will happen if not enough energy (carbon/carbohydrate) is available in the form of "groceries" (feed) the cow takes in. Usually the cow will rapidly lose condition and become skinny, which will reduce the potential milk yield. This is the well-known "milking the fat off the back" condition, since body reserves can be broken down by the liver into usable energy. But if this goes on too long and if the cow is not offered enough food to make up for the energy being drained out of her as harvestable milk twice daily, the cow's internal mechanisms will look for other forms of energy to utilize, such as fat, and the cow will then develop ketosis.

Ketosis is a condition in which cows are not taking in enough energy in their feed to balance their metabolic needs and then mobilize their body stores of fat, converting them to ketones in the liver. Theoretically, the animals are starving—starving for energy (carbohydrates in the form of sugars). The brain, which runs on glucose (sugar), *always* gets fueled first; if not, nothing else can occur. If the animal is not taking in enough energy to meet its needs, fat can be mobilized from body reserves and the liver can convert this fat to an energy source for the brain, albeit a less-than-ideal one—ketones. The brain can use this alternative source temporarily, but if it's used for a longer period the cow may develop nervous ketosis, a condition where the animal starts to acts crazy (more on this in a bit).

Ketosis can either be primary or secondary. Primary ketosis is the condition caused by the cow failing to take in enough energy, as described previously. Secondary ketosis is still ketosis but results from some other principal cause, most commonly a twisted stomach (displaced abomasum) or any condition where the cow is not taking in enough feed to meet its metabolic needs. Unfortunately primary ketosis itself can cause a twisted stomach. Ketosis also can lead to other problems, such as fatty liver and cystic ovaries. In older cows, where there is likely an underlying lack of calcium in the blood stream, especially when fresh, with associated poor digestive function, secondary ketosis can also be a problem. There are three types of ketosis: clinical ketosis, subclinical ketosis, and nervous ketosis.

Clinical ketosis is pretty well known: typically the cow is a bit depressed and almost sleepy-looking and walks around looking kind of "spacey," with her head slightly held up. She will eat mainly hay. Her manure will be firm and dry (approaching the appearance of horse manure), and she will have a sweet smell of ketones on her breath and in her milk (like nail polish or glue). Often, one can hear her heartbeat just behind the last rib on the left (rumen side) if listening with a stethoscope. And her urine will turn a Ketostick purple within a few seconds. Ketosis most frequently occurs in the first few weeks of lactation due to the strong demands for energy to make rapidly increasing amounts of milk. At first, you will see a gradual drop in milk production, and the cow will start to back off on her grain or energy feed (which is odd because that is what she needs). When surgically opening up a cow to fix a displaced abomasum, the same ketotic smell will come from within the opened abdominal cavity. While most ketosis occurs within the first month of calving, if a pregnant cow goes off-feed for whatever reason she can become ketotic since the calf requires lots of energy late in pregnancy. Thus, it is extremely important to examine off-feed dry cows or near-fresh cows and determine the cause. Again, low calcium can easily be a factor, especially in older cows.

I think by far the most common type of ketosis is subclinical ketosis, which can occur in the cow while you are happily milking her and feeding her without even realizing that she is borderline or slightly low in energy (blood sugar). Subclinical ketosis doesn't show the same visible symptoms as clinical ketosis. It can only be detected by using a urine strip or milk powder that detects low levels of ketones. I believe that a very high majority of fresh cows grazing in the spring have subclinical ketosis, robbing farmers of valuable production and reproductive capability. The biochemical Beta-hydroxy butyrate (BHB) is elevated in cows developing ketosis or that will develop ketosis. Commercial tests for BHB levels are available and should be used to predict ketosis in the near future and thereby closely monitor feed intake and give supportive care with energy supplements to prevent ketosis from occurring. If ketosis has been an issue, it is wise to test cows for BHB levels prior to calving.

If clinical ketosis is left untreated, the cow's brain can utilize ketones for only so long until she starts acting crazy. Once she starts nibbling at herself, gnawing at the pipes near her, or falling over, time is of the essence to get an IV of dextrose into her due to her dangerously low blood glucose levels. The bizarre signs a cow displays with nervous ketosis take about twelve hours to go away once treated with IV dextrose. If a cow is not treated with IV dextrose, she will become a downer cow with a poor prognosis for recovery. When combining signs of a down cow with bizarre behavior, the other diagnosis that rises to the surface is rabies, something we don't want to ever have to consider unless absolutely necessary.

Treatment

The treatment for ketosis is straightforward. The aim is to increase the cow's blood sugar. Administering 500cc dextrose IV will immediately increase the blood glucose levels to within normal; however, this will only last about four to six hours before blood glucose levels will decline again unless the cow starts to eat and take in her own energy. Providing an oral source of ingredients that the cow can convert to usable energy is the best way to help a cow get over ketosis. A follow-up and very appropriate treatment in the conventional dairy sector is propylene glycol, a three-carbon compound, given orally, eight ounces (one cup) twice daily as needed. This is like adding wood to the woodstove because the rumen can convert propylene glycol to carbohydrate sugars, which then enter the bloodstream of the cow. Then the liver won't be under stress to convert fats to energy.

But propylene glycol is not allowed for organics. Instead glycerin, another three-carbon compound, may be used if mixed with dextrose and labeled as "dextrose with glycerin as a carrier." Cows dislike the taste of propylene glycol but enjoy glycerin. Taste each for yourself and you'll see why. Using molasses or other sweet-tasting sugary compounds are also popular. Liver tonics such as LivWell with celandine, redroot and goldenseal or formulas with dandelion, and milk thistle would support liver function as would homeopathic

THE TREATMENT FOR KETOSIS IS STRAIGHTFORWARD. The aim is to increase the cow's blood sugar.

lycopodium and chelidonium (derived from celandine). A good practice is putting molasses on the feed so that the cow will be enticed to eat what is in front of her, instead of only forcibly giving it to her orally as a drench.

If you do want to drench a cow with molasses, a good drench would be a fifty-fifty mix of molasses and apple cider vinegar, fed at the rate of eight ounces of the mix twice daily as needed. Always hold the head just above parallel to the ground but *never* nose to sky since having the nose sky-high will more easily get liquids into the windpipe and lungs. When drenching anything, give the cow a little bit, stop to let her cough or spit it out a little, then drench some more, stop again, and so forth. *Never* just pour something into a cow's mouth without a care about how fast it goes in.

Prevention

A preventive technique against ketosis is to use choline (a B-like vitamin) in the pre-fresh ration. This has been shown to help the liver process low-density lipoproteins so they don't accumulate and result in fatty liver. Heavy, overconditioned cows *should* receive this in their pre-fresh ration. It is commercially available from Balchem as ReaShure, a rumen-protected choline that will not degrade immediately in the rumen but will pass into the small intestine and then be absorbed into the portal vein to the liver. Organic producers generally can use this product (but check with your certifier first). Alternatively, they can use 20cc intramuscular injections of choline chloride (Methaplex) once daily for five days just before freshening.

Preventing ketosis is obviously critical in order to get a good start in lactation as well as getting the cow bred back in a reasonable amount of time, since skinny, negative energy–balance cows tend not to get bred back easily. The whole idea, therefore, is to graze wisely and provide energy in the diet that the cow wants to eat and that is healthy for her. The best way is to fertilize the soil so that the pasture contains high-energy plants. A rough estimate of plant sugar can be obtained by taking a Brix reading. Squeeze a few drops of plant sap onto a refractometer. Looking into the refractometer, you will see a division between blue and white along the numbers. The point where blue meets white is the Brix level. The higher the better. The line can be very clear or fuzzy—the fuzzier the line, the higher the calcium content of the plant, which is a good thing. Always try to take a Brix reading later in the day since sugar production in a plant is directly related to photosynthesis (as well as the minerals available from the soil for enzymes in the plant's biochemical reactions).

Simply throwing grain at a skinny cow is a bad way to make up for lack of energy intake and can have disastrous consequences, especially during lush pasture growth, as rumen acidosis can occur due to insufficient intake of effective fiber relative to grain. Try to have a lot of clover in your pastures since clover provides energy (and cows love clover). Also try to graze paddocks at the height you would like to make good hay (clover at eight inches, alfalfa at about twelve to fourteen inches, or early bloom and grasses no later than early seed formation) since this will provide effective fiber to slow down the passage of feed in the rumen while still being nicely palatable. Too often people graze very young growth, which will hurt paddock regrowth and also fail to provide effective fiber to the rumen. The longer you can keep feed in the rumen (with structural fiber), the better the chance that the cow can extract its full nutritional value.

While the lower gut definitely also extracts nutritional value from feed, if there is not enough effective fiber in the rumen to slow feed passage, you will have too much "pasture manure" and lose nutrients out the back end. You can also run the risk of having grain pass from the rumen undigested and become fermented in the abomasum or the intestine, creating excess gas (in the abomasum) and low pH (in the intestine) where it should not. While dry hay is the best feed to slow down rumen passage, prevents acidosis and also helps create milk butterfat due to the acetic acid it produces in the rumen (and needing to chew cud more which offsets low pH), cows don't usually want to eat dry hay with the fresh green feed available in the paddocks. However, during pasture season, cows do still like to eat corn silage. And while many graziers do not want to feed corn silage, it has energy buried in it and does keep body condition on grazing cows, which is extremely im-

portant for them to avoid developing ketosis. Another feed cows will
also eat during grazing season is baleage, but it often has more protein
than energy, which does nothing to help prevent ketosis. In fact, baleage usually has high levels of soluble protein that, when added to the
diet of cows eating fresh pasture, compounds the problem of excess
protein in relation to energy.

Many cows get borderline ketosis. Whether you detect it is another
question. Just remember that ketosis is a thief—it robs your cow of her
energy and vitality, which can cause other serious problems. Feed your
cows well, keeping in mind that you have a large living mammal that
needs to nourish her basic metabolic processes, her growth, and her
udder for the milk you are removing. If you don't feed her correctly,
she will deplete her body and become a rack of bones that will have
trouble conceiving for months on end. Do whatever it takes to balance
the cow's biological requirement for energy and protein during the
grazing season. Monitoring body condition and milk urea nitrogen
(MUN) will ensure healthy grazing animals.

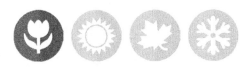

CHAPTER 4

Pasture and Grazing Systems

W hen spring is in the air, life unfolds in its many forms. The grass is lush and growing fast, and the cows are enjoying it. Crops are being planted, and some early crops are already being harvested. These are the crops that we intend to feed to the cattle as their primary source of nutrition for the time of year when green plants are no longer growing. But during mid-spring through early autumn, we should be thinking of pasture as the main feed. Why? For one, it's inexpensive. But more importantly, pasture is the healthiest feed due in part to the bovine digestive enzymes present in the gut and because grazing makes the cows exercise by moving around to harvest it. Perhaps even more importantly, it provides a diverse diet, which the cows appreciate—wouldn't you?

Grazing Systems

First, what is a grazing system? According to Edward B. Rayburn at the West Virginia Extension Service, a grazing system is "the combination of pastures, livestock, fences, and management used to control forage production and harvest. The development of a grazing system should be flexible and dependent on the livestock producer's goals and resources."* This definition is apt, for it takes into account that every farm will have a different grazing system; indeed, there is no one perfect grazing system. Depending on your needs, your grazing system can be high–milk production oriented, using pasture to supplement indoor feeding; medium- to high milk–production oriented, using increased pasture and less feed inputs in the barn; or low milk production–oriented, using the most possible pasture for dry matter intake. Well-managed intensive grazing systems have been shown to be a viable alternative to remain competitive for farmers. Since there'll be lower production per animal and lower income, farmers using grazing systems often increase their herd size and make needed improvements to improve pasture resources.

While "any cow knows how to eat grass," grazing does *not* mean less management. Actually grazing takes just as much true management as does total confinement herds to be successful. However, for those of you who do not now utilize existing pasture to its fullest extent, even if it's putting forty cows on only five acres, there are some things that you can still do to make sure that the pasture will provide as much possible feed throughout the grazing season as possible. For starters, break up any area of continuous pasture (also known as set-stocking) into smaller areas (paddocks). Try one-acre paddocks, divided up by single-strand polywire, and keep the cows on them for one to two days. You will need a source of water and a water line—a fifty-gallon trough is easy to dump out and move with quick couplers from your main water line to the water tubs. Clip pastures three days after grazing to splatter out manure paddies (this is free fertilizer) to kill the worm larvae. Waiting three days before disturbing the manure paddies allows dung beetles to drill what they will of the manure into the soil. If you're not used to grazing much and don't have a lot of dedicated pasture, this is a good place to start. The cows will like having some fresh greens to eat and the pasture will be rested to some degree to allow for regrowth prior to the animals grazing it again.

---

* http://www.caf.wvu.edu/~forage/grazing_sys.htm

Costs and Production

Granted, cows that are intensively grazed do not make as much milk in general if pasture makes up the vast majority of daily feed, but the feed costs are much lower. The cost of pasture as a nutritional component of the diet is generally accepted to be about one to three cents per pound of dry matter, whereas the cost of totally feeding in the barn is generally six to seven cents per pound of dry matter. A typical cow will eat about forty to forty-five pounds of dry matter daily, so the cost is $0.40–$1.20 for pasture if feeding 100 percent pasture whereas the cost per day will be about $2.40–$2.80 per day if feeding all stored feeds in the barn (not including any minerals or other supplements). Obviously cost of feed, whether produced on-farm or bought, can vary widely between farms and different regions, but the difference between cost of feed directly from pasture versus bringing stored feed to cows generally holds. Regardless of milk prices, a cheap source of feed to supplement some barn feeding seems worthy of consideration. A study that was conducted in the early 2000s by Tim Fritz and Beth Grove (both former extension agents) comparing the costs and income of different farming systems among the Amish farming community of Lancaster, Pennsylvania, showed that the most profitable were grazing farms that achieved a herd average of 21,000 pounds of milk per year—which happened to also be the average production for the 1,900 dairy farms in Lancaster County. This production level is an obtainable goal—if one is feeding his cows correctly both out on the pasture *and* in the barn. The comparison study did not look at the economics of organic production, which can allow for lower production levels while maintaining the best profitability levels due to higher prices for organic milk. I would highly recommend that anyone grazing should be consulting with a nutritionist who understand grazing systems and agrees with the philosophy of grazing in general.

Healthy Milk

For farmers only recently considering grazing , I can predict with near certainty that cow health will improve during the grazing season compared to cows kept inside all the time. Why? Mainly due to the fresh vegetation, but also because of the exercise. Exercise is very beneficial to fresh cows that haven't cleaned properly because it allows their lymphatic system to drain away problematic substances. A study I conducted as a summer project in Holland while in veterinary school showed that there were significantly less inflammatory conditions in cows on farms that practiced intensive grazing versus cows kept inside and fed diets of high amounts of ensiled feeds and grains.

The topic of conjugated linoleic acids (CLAs) and omega-3 fatty acids is an important one, since CLAs are a known and proven anti-carcinogen (cancer fighter). And it just so happens that grazing cows (and all grazing animals for that matter) have higher levels of CLAs and relatively more omega-3s than omega-6s than their grain-fed cousins confined to indoors. Omega-3s are anti-inflammatory. Exact levels need to be determined by getting the milk tested. There are also other beneficial short-chain and long-chain fatty acids in milk, as well as some medium-chain and trans-fatty acids (the bad fatty acids that can increase dangerous low-density lipoproteins). It all depends on what the cows are being fed.

One study from Australia on the effect of daily pasture intake on the concentration of CLA in milk fat when no concentrates were fed showed that CLA content increased as pasture intake increased. At pasture intake of 1.5 kilograms dry matter per cow per hundred kilograms live weight, there was 1.0 gram CLA per hundred grams of milk fat, while a pasture intake of 4.5 kilograms dry matter per cow per hundred kilograms live weight yielded 1.8 grams CLA per hundred grams of milk fat. The researchers found that, in general, the CLA concentration in the milk fat of grazing cows may be two to five times that of cows fed total mixed rations (TMR).*

The cis-9, trans-11 form of CLA is the most common form present in milk and is an intermediate compound of the metabolism of linoleic acid by the rumen bacterium *Butyrivibrio fibrisolvens*. Changes in feeds—such as different pasture species of grasses or alfalfa, different

---

* Stockdale et al., "Influence of Pasture and Concentrates in the Diet of Grazing Dairy Cows on the Fatty Acid Composition of Milk," Journal of Dairy Science 70 (2003): 267–76.

hays, and concentrates—and the extent of metabolism in the rumen affect the CLA concentration in ruminant products. Since bacteria change the cis-11 of linoleic acid to the trans-11 of CLA in the rumen, the amount CLA in the milk depends on both the levels of linoleic acid in the feed and how long the feed stays in the rumen. As pasture intake increases, the amount of time feed stays in the

And it just so happens that grazing cows (and all grazing animals for that matter) **HAVE HIGHER LEVELS OF CLAs AND RELATIVELY MORE OMEGA-3s** than omega-6s than their grain-fed cousins confined to indoors.

rumen decreases because the fresh, lush feed lacks effective structural fiber. Dry hay provides effective structural fiber, which slows down digestion. Quicker flow through the rumen may reduce the extent of metabolism, which would result in higher concentrations of CLAs. In other words, complete metabolism when linoleic acid remains in the rumen too long will result in milk with lower CLA content. Increasing an animal's pasture intake will thus decrease the amount of time the linoleic acid stays in the rumen and increase the CLA concentration in the ruminant's milk. (But manure may be very loose!)

Stockdale sums up his study in this way: "The results suggest that feeding cows plenty of good quality pasture with minimal quantities of cereal grain–based concentrates will result in milk with the healthiest fatty acid profiles." Basically, this study implies that grazing cows in normal body condition are healthiest and will yield the healthiest milk for consumers.

So, is it wise to know the quality and quantity of pasture your grazing cows are consuming? You bet it is.

NOP Pasture Rule

Have you been keeping track of your cows' pasture intake? Do you know yet if they are getting a minimum of 30 percent dry matter intake on average? Are you even keeping track of such things? Do you have any idea of what your cows are eating in terms of dry matter from all possible sources? If you are a certified organic dairy farmer in the United States, you *must* keep track of what you are feeding to your young weaned heifers, bred heifers, lactating cows, and dry cows in accordance with the USDA National Organic Program organic pasture regulations. Keeping track of your feed inventory will help you plan better, anyway.

Organic farms must graze animals six months of age and older for a minimum average of 30 percent dry matter intake from pasture over the grazing season for a minimum of not less than 120 days. The USDA National Organic Program (NOP) is serious about this regulation; failure to comply will result in decertification.

Complying with government rules unfortunately usually means keeping written records to prove that you are doing what you say you are doing. This is definitely the case for the pasture rule. How much stored feed (on a dry matter basis) have you been feeding your cows prior to turn out this year? How much are you feeding now? If you have accurate records and also use a TMR mixer (with functioning weigh scale), you can easily write down how much is being fed in the barn during the winter minus what is being fed in the barn during the summer, and you have a fairly quick and simple idea of pasture intake via this "back-calculation" method. This back-calculation assumes the cows are eating in the pasture what you are no longer feeding in the barn (everything figured on a dry matter basis). However, if body condition suffers greatly, there is a real likelihood that the cows may not be meeting their basic dry matter intake for the day (and therefore are losing body condition/weight). After all, if you are harvesting from them twice a day, they need to be replenished by the right amount of feed (from all sources) to maintain their basic biological needs, to carry a calf, and to make milk.

You should keep close track of which paddocks your cows, dry cows, bred heifers, and weaned heifers are in every single day, for how long, and the size and shape of the paddocks. Your certifier could ask you for such basic things at your next inspection. Having a large map of your pasture fields posted in the barn's office will let you quickly jot down when your milking herd is in what field. You can easily take a digital photo of such a map, which will then meet the requirement for record keeping of pasture usage.

In my area of Pennsylvania where livestock density is very high and grazing acreage is relatively low, it might be a good idea to learn how much dry matter is in your pasture. Once you get a feel for how much dry matter exists in your pastures, you can size individual paddocks appropriately for the amount of cows you plan to put in there for a twelve- or twenty-four-hour period. Moving cows every twelve hours is best as the cows enjoy fresh pasture after every milking and if you back fence them off what was grazed, that area will start regrowing more quickly than if they continue to trample it. Knowing how much dry matter is *available* to eat when your cows enter a paddock will help use paddock space the most efficiently as well as make sure you know what your animals are eating in terms of pasture dry matter intake. It's not a difficult process, and I have done this on many farms in various states. Having this kind of information will help you more accurately predict and then calculate what your cows are taking in from pasture.

You should also want to know how good your pasture is in terms of nutrition for your animals. You most likely already take hay, silage, and baleage samples—pasture sampling is also needed. A part of taking samples lately has been to get immediate Brix readings at the time of getting a pasture sample to send off to the lab for more in-depth analysis. Brix is an estimate of sugars in the plants that your animals will be eating. The sugars that a plant makes are directly tied to the amount of photosynthesis taking place. Brix can vary from day to day as well as time of day within the same plant. Therefore taking Brix readings later in the afternoon on sunny days will give a higher reading than early in the morning or on cloudy days. The refractometer reading measures dissolved solids in a couple drops of the plant sap. Thus, not only sugars are being measured but also minerals. The higher the number, the better. One study showed that cows making a certain amount of milk, fed a certain amount of grain, and grazing a low-Brix pasture could be fed much less grain when they were changed to pastures with higher Brix readings. That is money saved in paying out for grain and having healthier animals since they are getting their sugars/carbohydrates in a form that's very bioavailable and friendly to the gut. How do you get higher Brix readings? Mainly by adding the correct forms of calcium, sulfur, and boron as well as other necessary minerals to the soil. Having a healthy, balanced soil release minerals into the root zones will create more vigorous growing plants that can deliver more of what your animals will thrive on. A nutrient-rich, high-forage diet that you grow is smart business.

Nutrient and Energy Needs, Soluble Protein, and MUN
I think we can all agree that cows and other ruminants were created to eat fresh grass and other forages as their primary feed source. It is unfortunate that modern dairy farming constantly tries to divorce itself from this most basic concept by keeping cows confined inside and feeding relatively grain-rich rations that push high milk production at the cost of risking chronic low levels of rumen acidosis. However, even in pasture feeding systems, rumen acidosis is possible when only feeding lush pasture and then feeding slugs of grain at milking time, with ensiled grass baleage as the only other feed. I have seen it on a few farms. Try to get dry grass hay into your animals about half an hour prior to sending out. If they refuse to eat hay, add molasses on top of it to make it more inviting. The molasses and hay are very beneficial to a grazing animal in that the molasses will add energy to their diet and improve the internal carbon-to-nitrogen ratio. Cows also use energy by walking. The farther they walk to get to a paddock, the less energy they have to make milk.

Excess soluble protein (found in lush pasture and baleage) in the rumen is converted into urea by the liver but results in high blood urea nitrogen (BUN) and milk urea nitrogen (MUN). BUN can be turned into urine and excreted, while high MUN is excreted in the milk. But this excess protein nitrogen being converted to urea to be eventually excreted costs the animal biological energy (real energy that takes away from milk production). High levels of BUN, most easily reflected by evaluating levels of MUN in the milk during DHIA test day, can also sometimes interfere with reproduction. Good MUN levels are 8-12. Additionally, when the carbon-to-nitrogen ratio is too low (meaning too much nitrogen from protein), cows tend to get skinny. That is why I like to see decent body condition on cows coming out of the winter months heading into the new pasture season; they will likely lose condition due to the excess protein from pasture in relation to energy. That's the biology of the situation. Fine-tune your cows' ration to keep enough energy in it by talking wih your nutritionist.

Dry grass hay serves two purposes: to keep pasture bloat from occurring and to slow down the passage of ingested feed through the animal. If your grazing cows pass manure with ease, like a garden hose that just got turned on, then they are not absorbing as much of their feed as they could be. Alfalfa hay produced in the West—sometimes called "candy" hay in the East—will not help slow down the rate of passage as there often is "shatter" of the leaves snapping off the stems when dry and brittle, with the cows only eating the leaf and not the stalks, therefore not deriving any real fiber benefit from that hay. In addition, Western "candy" hay has too much protein to be feeding it during the springtime. By feeding medium-quality hay with molasses on it (so the cows will eat it), you are not only providing energy (the molasses) but also effective fiber. Cows really don't need to be pouring out thick, pea soup–like manure when on pasture. If they are, you are not getting efficient absorption of pasture nutrients they are simply running through the rumen extremely fast and not helping with the cow's basic metabolic and body conditions.

A healthy grazing animal that has a balanced ration is *not* skinny and shooting manure out the back end but rather is a sleek and fit athlete with a glossy coat. These animals will more often than not have good rumen fill. Rumen fill can be gauged by looking at the area behind the large ribs when the cow's head is to your left and her tail to your right. You should *not* see a caved-in upside down triangle—if you do, the animal has not eaten enough in the last six hours. If this remains the same over days and weeks, she will not make as much milk as she could have had she been fed more feed. If you are doing artificial insemination, you may want to keep feeding corn silage (if you grow that on your farm) throughout the grazing season to keep condition on the cows so they show a decent heat on which to breed. Feeding 20–30 pounds of corn silage year round is a good amount and will deliver about 3–5 pounds of grain within it.

Grain

So how much grain to feed to grazing cows? Well, first it needs to be said that when cows are fed grain, they will reduce their DMI from pasture. Or, to put it differently, if there's not enough DMI from pasture, they will gladly eat offered grain to meet their needs. First, don't feed more than twenty pounds of grain in a day to your highest producers (Holsteins making a hundred pounds of milk or more) and

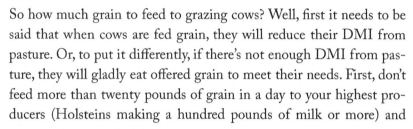

While most of this chapter is based on my own experience and thoughts, as my writing usually is, this next small part is taken right out of literature, just to give an idea of possible grain mixes. From F. B. Morrison's *Feeds and Feeding* (1949),

> When grazing cows was an integral part of dairy farming, a 12% protein grain mix is for cows on *excellent* pasture: (A) Ground corn 1160 lbs, ground oats 500 lbs, wheat bran 200 lbs, soybean oil mean or cottonseed meal 120 lbs, salt 20 lbs (makes 1 ton) or (B) Ground corn 1130 lbs, ground oats 500 lbs, wheat bran 200 lbs, linseed meal 150 lbs, salt 20 lbs. or (C) Ground barley 1030 lbs, ground oats 700 lbs, wheat bran 250 lbs, salt 20 lbs.
>
> A 14% protein grain mix for a *very good* pasture would be (A) Ground corn 1055 lbs, ground oats 500 lbs, wheat bran 200 lbs, soybean oil meal 225 lbs, salt 20 lbs, or (B) Ground corn 980 lbs, ground oats 500 lbs, wheat bran 200 lbs, linseed meal 300 lbs, salt 20 lbs. or (C) Ground barley 1090 lbs, ground oats 600 lbs, wheat bran 200 lbs, soybean oil mean or cottonseed meal 90 lbs, salt 20 lbs. Use a salt like Redmonds, loaded with trace minerals.

Notice in the information from Morrison's Feeds and Feeding that corn and barley were never in the same mix, not even at the 20 percent protein level (not shown), probably because of possible rumen acidosis occurring.

ideally spread it out over four feedings if possible—not just two slugs twice a day at milking because that risks rumen acidosis. If you are feeding corn silage into the summer, reduce the amount of grain fed since corn silage is part grain itself. If you feed corn silage, keep it to no more than thirty pounds per day. Generally the following guideline from Penn State applies:[*]

Production	Spring		Summer		Fall	
	lb.	G:M*	lb.	G:M	lb.	G:M
>80	20	1:4–1:5	22–24	1:3	20	1:4–1:5
70	15–18	1:4–1:5	19–21	1:3.5	16–18	1:4–1:5
60	11–13	1:5	15–18	1:4	12–14	1:5
50	8–10	1:5–1:6	10–12	1:4.5	8–10	1:4–1:5
<40	6–8	1:6–1:7	8–10	1:5	6–8	1:6–1:7

*G:M = grain:milk ratio

A completely alternative method is to feed an equal amount of grain to every cow regardless of stage of lactation. Between 2005 and 2010 many organic farmers averaged twelve pounds of grain per cow, some feeding a range with more grain to high producers and less to lower producers. After 2010, when organic grain prices kept going up, many producers reduced to an average of eight pounds of grain per cow. During this time period people started feeding a fixed amount of grain per cow regardless of stage of lactation. If you're willing to accept a lower peak milk, reduced body condition of fresh cows, and potentially lengthened time until first service, feeding equal amounts of low levels of grain is possible. Interestingly, at the same time, increasing consumer demand for grass-fed, grain-free milk opened up new markets for farmers. Disgusted at the ever-increasing cost of organic grain, partly fueled by competition from organic poultry growers that require grain to feed their birds, many organic grazing farmers have switched to grain-free grass-fed management systems. If studies continue showing that grass-based, grain-free milk is healthier for the

[*] Assume 1,300 pounds body weight. Guidelines are based on high-quality grass pasture available in adequate quantities.

human digestive system, the grain-free, grass-based dairy sector will undoubtedly flourish.

Dry Matter Available and Sizing of Paddocks

How do we know what amount of green, growing masses of edible plants are there for the animals once they arrive in a pasture field? Is there as much as you think? Might there actually be more? Or possibly less than you thought? How will you really know? The question is this: are you providing the right amount of pasture space to match what the paper ration says that they are eating in pasture? Are you giving them more space than what is needed—and therefore cheating yourself out of possibly making extra hay for winter time use? Instead of guessing or giving some repetitive, set amount of new area as you unwind the polywire, how about placing the polywire so you actually are giving the cows the right amount of space to match the planned dry matter intake?

Pasture is cheap feed because it is harvested by the cows themselves. They also fertilize the land. Matching what is standing there to what you desire your cows to take in from it will often result in spare acreage for you to mechanically harvest feed for later use—therefore less purchased feed needed. Even if sizing paddocks for 100 percent dry matter intake from pasture (like for growing heifers), I find most groups of animals are given *way* too much area. That wasted area could become hay or baleage! While there is a lot to be said about having nice amounts of room for exercise in a pasture, the mere fact that the cows are walking back and forth to pasture reduces the need for extra space for wandering about. However, if you have a herd of cows that still have their horns, you will indeed need some extra space since horned cattle do not like to be crowded for long periods of time. My friends David and Edie Griffiths, who have owned a biodynamic herd for a long time, give two acres for their sixty cows. That is, they give three-fourths of that for twelve hours and then open up the last quarter acre so the animals have the entire two acres during the second twelve hours. It works well for them.

What is the easiest way to know how much pasture is actually out there, in real time, right now? It's pretty simple actually. You need three basic things: thirty minutes once a week or whenever you are deciding to put the cows into a new field area, a small battery-powered digital scale ($50), a collapsible yardstick with sides of one foot each ($5),

Clean Pasture

Okay, let's start to talk about calves on pasture. First, always try to have calves on "clean" pasture. Clean means that adult cows haven't been on it for a couple years, and neither have other calves. This is very difficult to do in practice on farms with a small land base. Therefore, at the very least do *not* follow adult cows immediately with younger animals as this not only increases parasite pressure on the young stock but also increase likelihood of Johne's transmission to the young stock if adults are carrying the germs that cause Johne's disease. Many people will clip pastures in order to splatter out manure pies so the parasites dry up in the sun and wind, as well as to give a uniform regrowth of the paddock as mentioned previously. If you do not like to clip pasture, then I would suggest that you have poultry and hogs to peck and root through the manure pies, which they absolutely will do. You could also follow with sheep or goats, as most internal parasites are species specific. Grazing horses or mules right after cows have been in a pasture will "mow" the pasture down to an even height quite quickly, even right up close to manure paddies. But make sure that the horses or mules are taken out of that pasture strip after twelve hours or they will quickly graze it down to the bare earth thanks to their having both lower and upper front teeth. However, horses and mules will not destroy the existing cow pies like clipping or having poultry or hogs rooting through them would. Still try to use only clean pasture for calves, but if really tight on land consider the above recomendations.

handshears, and a large Tupperware box. With these in hand, you can become an excellent manager of your land and grazing cattle. Without these, you may be giving them too much space and wasting your forage resources. How do I know this? By having clipped some two hundred–plus pasture samples and sizing paddocks for dairy farmers, I found it doesn't take much more than a small part of an acre every twelve hours for a fifty-cow herd to meet the 30 percent dry matter intake required.

How can you do this for yourself? Identify a field where the herd will be for the next seven to ten days and scout the standing vegetation looking for uniformity or diversity of height and thickness, then pick one average spot the cows will graze. Next, outline one square foot of the standing pasture by placing your collapsible yard stick on the ground. Clip this one-square-foot sample down to about three or four inches, since you don't want to graze the stand any shorter. Now weigh the sample (in ounces) on your digital scale. Next, multiply the ounces of fresh grass by 456 (or if weighing in grams multiply by 15.2) to get pounds of dry matter per acre from the one square foot sample of fresh pasture. These conversion numbers take into account 20 percent dry matter of fresh pasture and 80 percent utilization rate if moving cows into new paddocks every 12–24 hours. The utilization rate reflects pasture being trampled upon as well as urinated and defecated upon.

> It is safe to say that organic cows weighing about twelve hundred pounds will, on average, need about **FORTY-FIVE POUNDS OF DRY FEED PER DAY** (regardless of whether it's stored feed, fresh pasture, or cardboard).

Now we can figure out what size paddock we will need for a herd of animals. It is safe to say that organic cows weighing about twelve hundred pounds will, on average, need about forty-five pounds of dry feed per day (regardless of whether it's stored feed, fresh pasture, or cardboard). And for this example, let's exceed the organic minimum of 30 percent intake from pasture just a little, so let's shoot for 33 percent (a third) of their daily intake to come from pasture. Since 33 percent of forty-five pounds is fifteen pounds, then one cow will need fifteen pounds from pasture for the day. Now say we have an acre of standing vegetation, which we find to be 1,600 pounds dry matter per acre from our clipping and calculation done right then and there in the field.

Since we figured one cow needs fifteen pounds from pasture (33 percent of forty-five pounds total dry matter intake in a day), then that one cow put into that field of 1,600 pounds dry matter needs only 0.009 acres of that stand (fifteen pounds needed/1,600 pounds available = 0.009 acres area needed). Multiply that one cow by the herd of fifty cows and we will need 0.45 acres for twenty-four hours. And if the herd is moved up every twelve hours, they will need just 0.225 acre of that stand for twelve hours—for the entire herd. That's not even a quarter acre every twelve hours for an entire fifty-cow herd!

Now imagine if you had been moving up the same fifty cows to a completely new acre of that same stand every twelve hours, but you actually only needed to provide 0.225 acres to get the 33 percent dry matter intake. I would say first that you should've given yourself a whole lot more dry matter intake credit than you did. More importantly, you could have potentially saved standing vegetation for later use—either for more grazing or harvesting it for stored feed. By not truly knowing what was out there, you either didn't take enough credit for actual pasture intake and/or you were going through pasture at a faster rate than you needed to.

Now, let's look at that same 1,600-pound dry matter per acre pasture stand from a different angle. Now let's say the paper ration shows they're getting 60 percent dry matter from the field. What size paddock would that same fifty-cow herd need now from that same field? Take the same forty-five pounds dry matter intake that one cow needs in a day (from whatever source, green grass to cardboard) but now multiply that by 60 percent to account for the new increased intake from pasture. One cow will now need to consume 28.8 pounds from pasture (versus the 15 pounds as shown earlier for 33 percent dry matter intake). Next, we again divide the pounds from pasture needed by one cow (28.8 pounds) by the same 1,600 pounds that is standing

Grazing When It's Hot

If you are already committed to grazing in general, here are a few tips to keep in mind for the summer. During the hottest time of the year, regular cool-season grasses go dormant, more or less. One way to help them "jump" when a rain does come is to not let pastures be grazed down too short. By keeping the height *no less* than three inches, there will be enough plant mass available for rapid regrowth when moisture comes along during the hot spell.

As crop insurance (nongovernmental kind), plant sorghum sudan grass for July and August heat. Sorghum sudan grass is a warm-season grass that loves the heat. For a forty- to fifty-cow herd, three to four acres is all that is needed. Plant it during the last two weeks of May, but not much past the first week of June (in southeastern Pennsylvania). The soil needs to be about 60°F, and you should drill it in no deeper than half an inch deep. If the soil is too cold or the grass is planted too deep, it won't start out well. Try to "stagger" its planting: two acres one week and two acres in another ten days. Since it normally comes up so fast and lush, this will help to not let it get ahead of you and the cows. Generally no herbicide is needed if planted correctly because of its fast growth. It does not do well being planted into an existing crop. A seedbed needs to be properly prepared and the sorghum-sudan planted into it. Graze it when it is about eighteen inches or higher to avoid any possibility of prussic acid (though that seems to have been bred out of this plant). Sorghum-sudan can also be cut and ensiled and, if cut at the right time and ensiled properly, is at least equivalent corn silage in terms of energy content. It is also more digestible with more effective fiber than corn silage.

there, and now one cow will require 0.018 acres to take in 60 percent from pasture. Multiply that again by fifty cows, and you'll find that an increased paddock size of 0.9 acres (0.018 x 50) for twenty-four hours is now needed. For twelve hours, it'll be half that (0.45 acres). If you'd been giving them one acre every twelve hours, you again wouldn't have taken enough dry matter intake credit.

But now let's say you don't use a single-string polywire system—all you have is immovable barbed-wire fencing of one-acre paddocks. You also don't have a nutritionist or paper ration. For this example, let's say you like to move your fifty-cow herd into a new one-acre paddock every twelve hours. How much is that one acre providing for dry matter intake, given the same 1,600 pounds dry matter per acre in the stand to utilize? Those fifty cows can consume thirty-two pounds each from that one-acre pasture paddock (1,600 pounds available divided by fifty cows). They still need to take in forty-five pounds of feed daily, regardless of whether it's from pasture or cardboard. In this example they are now receiving 71 percent of their dry matter intake from pasture (thirty-two pounds from pasture divided by forty-five pounds needed from wherever). The 71 percent is the actual number that reflects what they are encountering and eating.

These examples are to show you that unless you walk out into your field and take a couple of simple one-square-foot representative samples to truly know how much "stuff" is standing there ready to be grazed, you could be wildly off in your thinking about how much dry matter intake your cows are receiving. For those using the "back calculation" method of simply taking the wintertime ration dry matter provided and then subtracting a springtime paper ration dry matter provided in the barn and thinking that the remainder is coming from pasture, please realize that you may be actually *shortchanging* yourself in actual dry matter consumed out on pasture. Taking a straightforward, real-life pasture sample(s) and weighing it is the simplest way you will ever come close to providing the correct space to reflect what you want the cows to be taking in. This method allows you to understand what paddocks provide in terms of dry matter intake and to better manage your pasture during dry times as well as lush growing times. So, for a $60 investment and thirty minutes a week, you can learn how to correctly balance what your cattle need with what the pasture provides.

Plants in Pasture

Walking to survey pastures is not only healthy exercise but also educational and empowering for you to manage a basic feed source more effectively. Walking through the areas where cows will be (or where they have been) reveals some interesting facts. First, it lets you recognize if a pasture is ready to be grazed or if it still needs rest time to grow more. Second, it shows you what they ate and how much they leave behind. Third, it shows you what they don't eat at all. Let's consider what they do eat. Warm-season annuals like sorghum-sudangrass—a lifesaver for the hot and humid weather of summer—is eaten well but somewhat unevenly, from a starting height of twenty to thirty inches down to about ten to twelve inches high. Orchard grass bunches that are about twelve to sixteen inches high are usually eaten evenly down to about five inches. Cows love clover, and if you start them on it at seven to eight inches high with blooms they will usually eat it fairly short, usually down to about three inches. Fescue, while it grows well during the heat when other cool-season grasses go dormant, is not a preferred feed it seems. It is very rough on the back side of the grass blade. They don't seem to eat it much, especially if other green feed is nearby. But it is good for autumn grazing as a frost will soften it up, making it much more palatable. Timothy is enjoyed by cows, but it's not as widespread anymore, at least in my region. Perennial rye grass is liked prior to it going to head, as with most grasses. Interestingly, if orchard grass goes to head, it will have a poorer taste (due to internal chemical changes) for the rest of the pasture season, even if you clip it after it's headed out.

There are other plants that cows will eat that are not necessarily planted as forages; hence, they are termed "weeds." Cows devour lambsquarters (*Chenopodium ambrosioides*) and the amaranth, smooth pigweed. Lambsquarters is generally high in calcium, as verified by a blurry line when taking a Brix reading from it. Burdock and dandelion are commonly eaten as well. I'm glad to see cows eat these "weeds" as they add diversity to their diet. In fact, they eat little bits of many other plants as they wrap their tongues around their main target or they may nibble at them at will if they are exposed to those species when

Individuality in Feeding Animals

As I look at the calendar on my wall, I see a picture of a boy walking in front of a long line of about a hundred cows eating a total mixed ration (TMR) at a feed bunk. While it can be easy to simply see the long line of cows as identical to each other in terms of a production unit, it is just as easy to see each and every animal as unique and individual from each other. Seeing the individuality of animals allows us to think beyond the simplistic view of group averages to realizing that each animal has specific nutritional needs. This concept is true whether we are looking at a herd of cows, a herd of goats or pigs, a flock of sheep, a band of horses, a pride of lions, or even a school of fish. Each animal will respond differently to the feed it is fed or finds because of different individual metabolic needs. Metabolic needs will differ upon each animal's genetic make-up as well as the stage of life.

A TMR is designed to perfectly feed only the perfectly average cow in the herd. While TMRs can provide a herd with a desirable forage-to-grain ratio, the minerals delivered will not be accurate to the needs for most cows. It isn't rocket science to realize that there is a quite a range of animals in a herd, varying in body size to different stages of lactation and pregnancy and growth. So if you have a herd of eighty cows with sixty-five Holsteins and fifteen Jerseys, it is rather obvious that each of their needs will be different. Add to this that some of each will be early lactation and climbing in milk production while others are past peak and some will have been recently bred while others are long bred, and it becomes very obvious that their mineral needs will vary greatly, yet the TMR delivers the same exact homogeneous mix of food and minerals to them all.

Some animals may need relatively more of one mineral than another. This would hold true for any mineral element. For instance, fresh cows need lots more daily calcium than cows ready to dry off. Calcium is tightly regulated in the bloodstream via the parathyroid gland, and we know that Jerseys have more problems keeping calcium in balance than other breeds. Zinc, needed for good hoof health, may be needed in different amounts for Holsteins with their white hooves than for Brown Swiss with their black hooves. Each animal will need different proportions of minerals in her diet than the next animal, yet the TMR delivers the same proportion day after day after day.

What am I trying to get at? Well, it seems to me that regardless of how smart (or not) you may consider cows, simply realizing that individuals will need and uniquely respond to what is in front of them makes sense. And, additionally, it has been proven that cows can select what they need by various internal bio-feedback mechanisms. It is well known that foraging animals will seek out what they need, sometimes in depraved ways: cows eating rabbits to get phosphorus they desperately crave, animals eating dirt to take in minerals that are lacking in the diet fed out to them, pre-weaned calves eating their bedding to get fiber because they are being denied hay until weaning, etc. It is also known that animals will select plant species that would seem to play no real part of their diet: calves eating burdock leaves, horses eating willow leaves, monkeys eating bitter, tannin-containing leaves, etc. In these cases they are self-medicating. How they sense what to eat is still a big mystery, but it is clear that they are drawn to certain things to satisfy deep urges. Call it intuition, call it instinct, call it whatever you will, but they are trying to tell us something: as individuals they can and do select what they want in their diet.

Therefore, maybe we should provide only the basics of the ration in a TMR so that the baseline of the animals is covered, but then rely more heavily on them to self-select what else they need, especially in terms of minerals. In practical terms, this would mean providing sources of free-choice minerals such as kelp, bioavailable sources of calcium, phosphorus, magnesium, zinc, bicarb, clay, and trace mineralized salt. Be prepared to watch some of the minerals disappear quickly. Be happy, for you have then allowed your animals to balance their own ration—and to tell you what your base ration may be lacking.

This same concept holds for pasture: try to have a biodiverse pasture. Having only one or two plant species (like white clover and perennial rye grass) in a pasture will not lead to a very balanced intake, whereas a pasture full of variety (and yes, "weeds") will allow animals to pick and choose to their heart's content. If you're worried about "weeds" being refused, please know that animals eating "weeds" should tell you something, for the "weeds" usually have quite a good mineral profile as many are somewhat deeply rooted or at least provide variety to the one or two plant species purposely planted for pasture intake. The only time I can see a monoculture being grown would be with a warm season annual like sorghum-sudan to germinate quickly and give vigorous growth during the heat when the native cool season plants aren't growing.

Providing diversity, both in plants and minerals, in the diet is a good thing, for it parallels both the diversity of individuals in a herd as well as allowing them to choose what they specifically want to eat. Diversity is the opposite of homogenization. Too many things in life seem to be "homogenized" these days. Isn't it ironic that individuality is both highly prized in our general society but also made bland by everyone buying the same stuff at the same chain stores? Being unique as God intended each of us to be is certainly good, right? Likewise, each animal is unique, an individual with individual needs—whether it is one of a line of a hundred cows at a feed bunk or individually named animals in a small, tie-stall herd. Each and every one of them has individual needs that can best be met by careful attention to correct feeding. Allowing animals themselves to select pasture plants and freely choose various minerals provided allow them to satisfy their own unique set of dietary needs.

the plant is young and green, perhaps early in the season when first let out to pasture and desiring lots of fresh green herbage. They don't eat much of thorny plants like horsenettle and cocklebur—plants with firm spikes on the underside of their leaves. Nor do they eat much bull thistle, Canada thistle, or spiny redroot pigweed; however, cows can be seen grazing the top seed heads of spiny redroot as well as the blooms of thistles. They don't seem to eat velvet leaf at all as that is almost always seen left intact and going on to seed. On a typical pasture in my area, I probably see about fifteen to twenty species of plants during my pasture walks, some of which I have yet to identify. Truly, walking your pasture will help you understand it much better, both from a management perspective as well as from the cows' perspective.

With sorghum-sudan, lambsquarters, and smooth pigweed, you need to be careful not to set animals on them right after the first rain following very dry conditions as these plants will take up nitrates and become temporarily toxic. Sorghum-sudan, though a wonderful forage for high summer, can also be temporarily toxic with prussic acid if grazed too young; however, the brown mid-rib varieties seem to have had that potential toxicity bred out of them as I see many herds grazing sorghum-sudangrass that is only twelve inches high.

Keep in mind, however, that truly toxic plants do exist. These include bracken fern, wild cherry leaves that are wilted, ergot growing upon rye during prolonged cool and damp weather, horsetail, horse chestnut, false hellebore, jimsonweed (thornapple), mountain laurel, common milkweed, horsenettle, deadly nightshade, wilted red maple leaves, pokeweed, oak acorns, white snakeroot, water hemlock, and the garden yew bush. Many grow in the hedgerows. For instance, in 2010 we saw a bumper crop of poison hemlock, which looks like Queen Anne's Lace but much taller and with purple spots on the stem. It was everywhere in roadside ditches and the perimeters of fields. Pokeweed begins growing quickly late in summer and develops its well-recognized smooth and shiny clusters of purple berries in about a month's time. Fortunately cows do not normally ingest poisonous plants when normal pasture species and "weeds" are available to graze.

By midsummer there is a lot of horsenettle growing. Horsenettle is easily found in pastures, growing to about eight to twelve inches high with small, white flowers with a yellow center; its stems and the undersides of leaves have small thorns. This is a poisonous plant, closely related to deadly nightshade. Deadly nightshade has small, dark-purple flowers and begins its vegetative growth in the spring (usually near fences and old wood piles). Jimsonweed, another poisonous cousin to horsenettle and deadly nightshade, is an easy-to-spot plant, growing to about three feet tall with large, trumpet-shaped, light-purple flowers.

I am a strong believer in clipping pastures to ensure good pasture management. I am not at all sure I believe in what people are calling "tall grazing" if it means letting all kinds of plants go to seed since cows like fresh, green, growing plants. In trying to get at the lower-to-the-ground green areas of older plants, animals increase their chances of getting pinkeye as they poke through rank, mature growth to get at the lush growth underneath—this makes their eyes water and attracts flies. If for no other reason, clipping will dramatically reduce the number of unwanted species taking over a pasture field. More importantly, clipping also allows uniform regrowth of your desired plants, allowing you to know when to put your cows back on a pasture. Sorghum-sudan can do an excellent job at regrowth when it is clipped, as it will be very uneven in height if unclipped.

For pastures with very uneven growth due to animals grazing around certain plants (not toxic but simply not as preferred), consider pre-clipping a field and letting the plants wilt. This will make everything more palatable to the animals, thus encouraging them to take in a true variety of plants (all green matter), and also reduce the bloat potential of legumes. Pre-clip anywhere from two to four hours before grazing. Pre-clipping can be done up to forty-eight hours prior to cows entering a pasture. But *do not* pre-clip pastures that contain truly toxic plants (another reason to walk your pastures regularly).

Herb Analysis Chart

	Alfalfa	Dandelion	Lamb's Qtr	Chicory	Comfrey	Plaintain	Nettle Leaf	Burdock	Cleavers
Protein	20.97%	25.00%	31.70%	19.5	23.7	19.6	25.7	29.0	11.7
Digestable Protein				14.7	18.5	14.7	20.4	23.5	7.3
Soluble Protein				4.7	2.7	2.9	4.3	3.9	1.2
Protein Solubility	50.07%	24.40%	18.10%	24.2	11.4	15.0	16.8	13.4	9.9
Nitrogen/Sulfur Ratio	11:1	10:1	12:1	8:1	14:1	6:1	4:1	5:1	7:1
Acid Detergent Fiber	32.10%	19.20%	15.00%	32.8	29.8	34.1	22.6	25.1	40.6
Neutral Detergent Fiber	43.61%	30.00%	21.90%	46.8	42.2	45.8	34.4	36.5	49.1
Relative Feed Value	136.20%	229.00%	329.00%	126	145	127	193	177	108
TDN* (est)	63.89%	80.90%	85.60%	63.5	66.8	64.4	74.5	71.8	57.1
ME (mcal/b)		1.33	1.41	1.04	1.10	1.06	1.22	1.18	0.94
Est.Net Energy (themstc wt)	0.65	69.9	74.3	54.0	57.0	54.7	64	61.6	48
NE Lact (mcal/b)		0.085	0.9	0.65	0.69	0.66	0.77	0.075	0.58
NE Maint (mcalb)		0.895	0.959	0.648	0.697	0.661	0.806	0.0768	0.551
NE/Gain (mcalb)		0.6	0.655	0.383	0.426	0.394	0.523	0.490	0.295
Calcium	1.58%	1.04%	1.10%	0.89	273	1.84	4.38	2.10	1.3
Phosphorous	0.37%	0.33%	0.39%	0.31	020	0.26	0.41	0.34	0.39
Potassium	2.05%	4.46%	7.66%	3.59	394	2.97	3.01	3.28	2.46
Magnesium	0.46%	0.26%	0.55%	0.26	0.39	0.17	0.39	0.43	0.25
Sodium	759ppm			0.04	0.04	0.04	0.011	0.005	0.014
Sulfur-total	0.31%	0.41%	0.43%	0.37	0.27	0.53	0.94	0.90	0.26
ppm Iron	171	657	91	195	176	83	349	149	70
ppm Copper	15	15	8	14	29	12	11	26	13
ppm Zinc	30	34	46	43	46	44	40	32	127
ppm Manganese	23	35	138	36	192	30	36	47	66
ppm Boron	50	30	44	28	42	29	67	32	15

	Alfalfa	DayLily Leaf	DayLily Blossom	Echinacea Leaf	Wild Grape Leaf	Wild Rasp Leaf	Willow Leaf	Hazlenut Leaf	Mulberry Leaf	Chinese Chestn Lf
Protein	20.97%	20.6	23.4	15.7	22.1	15.2	19.8	14.1	26.2	21.8
Digestable Protein		15.7	18.3	11.1	17.1	10.6	14.9	9.6	20.9	16.7
Soluble Protein		5.4	14.8	1.8	1.2	0.4	1.5	0.7	3.6	14.7
Protein Solubility	50.07%	26.4	63.0	11.4	5.6	2.8	7.5	4.9	13.7	67.7
Nitrogen/Sulfur Ratio	11:1	19:1	20:1	12:1	14:1	16:1	7:1	14:1	17:1	11:1
Acid Detergent Fiber	32.10%	28.2	17.0	20.0	19.5	22.6	24.9	20.2	21.5	41.2
Neutral Detergent Fiber	43.01%	35.7	23.5	29.3	34.6	43.1	37.6	42.3	43.2	70.9
Relative Feed Value	136.20%	175	299	233	198	154	172	161	197	75
TDN (est)	63.89%	70.9	83.4	77.3	77.8	74.5	72.0	77.1	75.7	54.6
ME (mcal/b)		1.16	1.37	1.27	1.28	1.22	1.18	1.27	1.24	0.9
Est.Net Energy (themstc wt)	0.65	60.7	72.2	66.6	67.1	64.0	61.8	66.4	65.1	45.7
NE Lact (mcal/b)		0.74	0.87	0.81	0.81	0.77	0.75	0.8	0.79	0.55
NE Maint (mcalb)		0.756	0.929	0.845	0.853	0.806	0.771	0.842	0.823	0.513
NE/Gain (mcalb)		0.479	0.629	0.557	0.564	0.523	0.493	0.555	0.538	0.259
Calcium	1.58%	0.81	0.39	2.57	1.91	0.85	1.45	1.44	3.09	1.37
Phosphorous	0.37%	0.25	0.43	0.25	0.32	0.16	0.23	0.12	0.26	0.2
Potassium	2.05%	2.24	2.17	2.22	0.95	1.6	1.71	0.75	1.85	0.84
Magnesium	0.46%	0.20	0.17	0.88	0.25	0.29	0.27	0.31	0.34	0.37
Sodium	759ppm	0.025	0.05	0.02	0.02	0.01	0.011	0.04	0.016	0.015
Sulfur-total	0.31%	0.17	0.19	0.21	0.25	0.15	0.44	0.16	0.24	0.31
ppm Iron	171	203	86	131	502	100	117	118	154	120
ppm Copper	15	10	22	21	16	18	13	19	12	15
ppm Zinc	30	25	66	32	32	35	105	27	36	61
ppm Manganese	23	54	40	132	89	210	101	373	63	160
ppm Boron	50	49	16	66	31	23	34	28	36	72

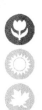

Source: Jerry Brunetti, Agri-Dynamics, used by permission.

Nutritious Weeds

Probably the best aspect to pasturing cows is that they can pick and choose from among a variety of live, growing plants, rather than only consuming a constant supply of stored, fermented feeds. The variety of plants that they will consume no doubt includes what people commonly call weeds. Yet I am no longer sure what the definition of a weed really is. The conventional definition is a plant growing where *we* don't want it to. But if animals eat it, then couldn't such a plant be considered a feed source? And what if the plant that is readily eaten also contains nutrients and phyto-chemicals that rival or exceed those found in alfalfa, ryegrass, or clover? Then the "weed" might even be considered beneficial to the cows' overall diet, providing both essential nutrients in addition to possible medicinal components.

In a 2006 study, pasture weeds analyzed on New Zealand's Massey University organic and conventional dairy farms showed that most of these "weeds" had the same or better feed quality (in terms of acid detergent fiber) as their perennial ryegrass and white clover stands, and higher macro- and micronutrients. In terms of macro- and micronutrients, chicory had significantly higher levels of P, S, Mg, Na, Cu, Zn, and B; narrow leaf plantain had higher levels of P, S, Ca, Na, Cu, Zn, and Co; and dandelion had significantly higher amounts of P, Mg, Na, Cu, Zn, and B.

A study by Jerry Brunetti of Agri-Dynamics in 2000 compared common weeds to alfalfa. In terms of macro- and micronutrients, nettle leaf showed better results than alfalfa in thirteen measurements: protein, nitrogen-to-sulfur ratio, acid detergent fiber, total digestible nutrients, net energy for lactation, Ca, P, K, S, Fe, Zn, Mn, and B. Dandelion was better in twelve measurements, comfrey in ten, and chicory and plantain in eight measurements compared to alfalfa.

An old study from 1933 in Oklahoma found that all the "weeds" tested were higher in nitrogen, phosphorus, and calcium than the native grasses and that young plants were higher in mineral nutrients and nitrogen than older plants. The researchers' overall conclusion was that "the presence of these weeds in the hay would increase the total mineral content of the forage, and under many conditions this effect would improve rather than injure its feeding value."

Secondary plant metabolites in fresh plants (pasture) can provide medicinal qualities, and animals instinctively search out plants that are high in condensed tannins, such as chicory, which help to repel internal worms—maybe they can sense this and actively seek them out. Then there are the nonbloating legumes with high tannins, such as birdsfoot trefoil, lespedeza, and sanfoin. All have shown to decrease internal worm burdens in live animal studies. The worms reduced are those that are common in weaned groups of heifers placed on the same pasture year after year—areas where parasites are just waiting for them time and time again.

I have observed that cows, heifers, and steers will readily eat nearly any and all forages and weeds but not truly toxic plants—if the plants are in a young stage of life. Once a plant starts going to seed, most animals won't eat them unless forced to (by starvation or simply nothing else to eat). From the old Oklahoma study that concluded young plants have more nutrients and the New Zealand and Agri-Dynamics study that showed which and how much of each nutrient is present, it is reasonable to state that having a true variety of plants in the pasture is beneficial for cattle.

> I HAVE OBSERVED THAT COWS, HEIFERS, AND STEERS will readily eat nearly any and all forages and weeds but not truly toxic plants—if the plants are in a young stage of life.

While you're out moving up fence, see what the cows have eaten in the last paddock. It'll most likely surprise you. It's fun to watch herbivores eating pasture and along the margins of laneways—and by their sleek hair coat, good muscle definition, and health stripes, you'll know that you are treating them well.

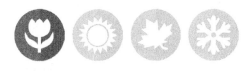

CHAPTER 5

Herbal Medicine

As plants green up in spring, it would be nice to know about medicines from plants. Fresh herbs, dried herbs, fluid extracts, tinctures, glycerites, extract tablets, and freeze-dried granules are all examples of botanical medicines, as are herbal teas and regular black tea for that matter. I believe there is good reason that cows, being herbivores, are well adapted to using botanical medicines very efficiently. Their ability to handle plants (and therefore plant-based medicines) is based on the activity of their bacteria and protozoa in the rumen and the digestive enzymes in the small intestine.

Evaluating Tinctures

Some farmers make their own tinctures at home and can discover what works best for themselves. Others choose to purchase tinctures from popular manufacturers, such as Herbal Vitality (where I purchase many of mine for work with cows), Gaia Herbs, Buck Mountain Botanicals, and Starwest Botanicals. When purchasing tinctures and dried herbs of commercial origin, keep in mind that the integrity of the manufacturer is paramount. Some websites and brochures present a clear picture of the manufacturing facility. Get a sense of the manufacturer's knowledge of plants and his educational background in the herbal world. Perhaps the manufacturer holds degrees or certificates to support assertions of natural plant medicine knowledge. Is the person interacting with peers in order to stay on the cutting edge? And perhaps most important, what do you sense and feel when talking with them on the phone or in person? Definitely read the entire label of any tinctures you buy. The following basics will help to identify a reputable manufacturer:

1. Use of proper name (i.e., *Echinacea angustifolia* vs. *Echinacea purpurea* vs. *Echinacea pallida*—which is in the bottle?). It matters, for each of these three different types of Echinacea provide differing amounts of plant compounds to the end product. If a label simply says "Echinacea," there is a chance that it is the least medically active or will not provide the amounts you are hoping for.

2. Strength of concentration (1:1, 1:3, 1:5, etc.). For example, 1:5 means that the manufacturer used one part herb for every five parts liquid. A 1:1 tincture is therefore stronger than a 1:5 tincture. However, real herbalists don't always use the strongest possible concentration; they often use the concentration that brings out the most balanced form of compounds. If a manufacturer does not state the concentration, be suspicious of unnecessary dilution to stretch raw material and therefore an unnecessarily weak formula.

3. Alcohol content. This has more to do with making sure that certain compounds are extracted and in solution. For instance, if you are getting an herbal medicine of barberry and would like the antibacterial berberines to be available, then a high alcohol content is necessary since berberine alkaloids can only be extracted at high alcohol levels (80 percent for alkaloids in general). Most common plant compounds can be extracted at much lower concentrations, like 25–40 percent, meaning that they are being extracted in 60–75 percent water. Interestingly, if you're using glycerin for extraction purposes, plant compounds that are extractable with water are equally extractable with glycerin. Glycerin is a sweet, syrupy substance that makes taking a plant medicine very easy, especially when dosing animals. Animals like sweet things just like we do. They re-

ally can't stand alcohol-based substances and will likely spit them out if given a chance or froth at the mouth as a cat will do before it gets sick to its stomach. A more folksy method is to use vinegar (apple cider or grape) for extraction. Technically, a glycerite or a "vinegarite" is not a tincture, just as a water extract is not a tincture since the word "tincture" means alcohol based. However, the term is generally applied to any liquid-based plant extract offered for sale. Whatever product type you end up liking to use, remember that alcohol extractions are the best preserved (longest shelf life).

4. Part of plant used (root, rhizome, herb, or flower). While beginners may not worry about which specific part of a plant is used, it can make or break the medicinal value of tincture. For instance, there is a huge difference between using the shoots or the bulbs of the garlic plant. While garlic is an obvious example, others may not be.

5. Whether fresh or dried material was used for extraction. Fresh herbs are always the best to use for extraction purposes, as a rule.

Some companies may not display the strength on the label, but they will then specify it in the catalogue (Starwest). If the strength is not specified on the label or in the catalogue, you have no idea how strong or weak of a tincture you are buying—but more importantly you won't know if it is being made consistently from batch to batch. The best plant medicines come from facilities current for Good Manufacturing Practices. This means that the facility keeps close track of where their raw ingredients come from and when and exactly how batches were made. Correct information is critical to successful and safe use of a product. Safety should come above all else; remember, *dose separates therapy from toxicity*. If you don't know the strength of the tincture, you cannot possibly know the correct dose to use. Perhaps more importantly, you may be wasting your money. To be sure, farmers can make their own tinctures, but try to at least have some training by a professional herbalist before relying on your products for medicinal use with your animals.

Next, please compare a few different manufacturers by inspecting a specific tincture of each—for instance, compare different garlic tinctures (*Allium sativum*). Hold up the tinctures to the light and inspect the depth of color. Generally the darker a tincture, the stronger it is. Open the bottle and smell the product for the richness of aroma. A well-made tincture should *not* smell like alcohol (or whatever base is being used). Most well-made tinctures of roots will have a strong, earthy aroma, while tinctures made from flowers will have a light and lifting fragrance. Lastly, taste it—if only to know what your animal patient will be experiencing. Is it agreeable or very bitter or sour? If bitter and sour, maybe it is best to put the dose on a sugar cube to administer it. My supplier at Herbal Vitality is a master herbalist and holds a PhD in experimental medicine. He creates the absolute strongest and most energetic tinctures I've come across—and for the same price as other popular brands. I would urge all readers to compare the tinctures you are using to at least one or two different brands to see what the differences are.

Administering Herbal Remedies

The most traditional method of administering tinctures and other herbal medicines (teas, dry herbs, tablets, etc.) is through the mouth. There are two good reasons for giving herbs orally. First, it is how an animal normally take plants into their system; its digestive tract is thus alerted and can respond, since it's biologically geared to take in plants anyway.

The second important reason to give herbal medicines by mouth is that the sense organs are very concentrated in the head area. The tongue's sense of taste is directly related to the nose's sense of smell, while our vision and hearing help orient us in space and time. These four senses are the primary physical senses of our herbivorous animal friends, as they don't have sensitive fingertips for touch like we do. The four main sense organs are only a very short distance away from the brain, which processes incoming information with amazing speed. Additionally, there are lymph nodes near the base of the tongue, behind the jaw, and along the throat that help process incoming information toward the immune system. Between the brain's immediate response to the herb via the facial senses and the digestive tract's ability to sift, sort, and absorb plant material, oral administration is easily the best method of giving herbal medicines—whether they be tinctures, essential oils, dried herbs, teas, or glycerites.

Even if given herbal medicine through methods other than by mouth, the entire herbivore system of the cow, sheep, goat, or horse should respond well. When I had read in the late 1990s that the Chinese give herbal teas to humans intravenously (IV) in hospitals, I knew I had to try it on my bovine patients. I've given tinctures IV since then (in dextrose) and am generally pleased with the results. However, you *must* make sure that the tincture is extremely well made if it's going directly into the blood stream. You should see *no* "snowflakes" suspended in the solution when looking at it after it is shaken.

While dosing is something of an art, there are volumes and volumes of work showing exactly how much of different tinctures to use for a variety of species. Veterinarians in the old days had detailed charts of how much of each tincture to use for cows, horses, pigs, sheep, dogs, and cats. There is no one dosage to give a cow for various tinctures—they are as varied as the pattern of spots on a Holstein.

The list of dosages shown below is a snippet from a book I stumbled upon many years ago; it's a gold mine of real information about plants used by veterinarians for animals "back in the day" when botanical medicine was commonly used by veterinarians. It's called *The Book of Veterinary Doses* by Dr. Pierre Fish.* Dr. Fish was dean of the Cornell Veterinary School from 1929 to 1931. *All doses shown are tinctures for oral administration in milliliters (cc).*

	Cow and Horse	Sheep and Pig	Dog
Aconite	0.2–6	0.25–1	0.13–0.5
Aloe	8–40	4–15	0.13–4
Arnica	15–30	4–8	0.6–1.3
Belladona	15–30	4–8	1–2
Bryonia	15–30	2–4	0.3–2
Calendula	15–30	4–8	1–2

* *Pierre Fish, The Book of Veterinary Doses, Therapeutic Terms and Prescription Writing (Ithaca, NY: Comstock, 1930). First published in 1904.*

	Cow and Horse	Sheep and Pig	Dog
Eucalyptus oil	8–15	1–3	0.3–1
Fennel	30–60	8–12	0.6–1.3
Ginger	30–60	8–15	0.6–4
Goldenseal	30–60	4–15	2–8
Licorice	15–60	4–15	0.6–4
Nux vomica	4–24	1.3–6	0.3–1
Peppermint oil	1–2	0.3–0.6	0.06–0.3
Pokeweed	4–8	1.3–3	0.3–2
Quassia	30–60	4–12	1–4
Thyme oil	2–8	0.3–2	0.06–1
Vinegar	30–120	2–8	1–4
Wintergreen	8–30	2–8	0.3–1

In their widely acclaimed 2007 book *Veterinary Herbal Medicine*, Dr. Susan Wynn and Dr. Barbara Fougère also show dosages of herbs to give. The doses shown in the table are from modern-day veterinary practitioners all over the world who use herbs. What's really nice is that these doses match up fairly well with the doses used in the 1930s, with the dose for tinctures being between 1–3 tablespoons, which is approximately 15cc–45cc total per dose (1 tablespoon = 15cc; 1 teaspoon = 5cc).

Preparation	Goat	Cow	Horse
Decoction (tea)	4 oz	12 oz	8 oz
Extract tablets	3–5	10–15	10–15
Freeze-dried granules	1 tsp	2 Tbsp	2 Tbsp
Tincture	1 tsp (5cc)	2 Tbsp (30cc)	2–3 Tbsp (30–45cc)

I am pleased to have both Dr. Wynn and Dr. Fougère as friends, and we're among the original members of the Veterinary Botanical Medical Association (VBMA), which was founded in 2002. The association is a worldwide group of veterinarians dedicated to using plant medicine with animals. My commitment to the VBMA is long-term and I am happy to say that the VBMA is working with the American Veterinary Medical Association to have duly trained and qualified veterinarians become board-certified specialists, much like, for example, orthopedic surgeons, radiologists and cardiologists already are. The VBMA promotes the science, traditional use, and energetic aspects of herbs. I invite you or any veterinarian you work with to learn from the VBMA website, www.vbma.org.

Jim Duke, the world-renowned botanist and retired USDA Agricultural Research Service researcher, has compiled a vast amount of information regarding herbs. The highest scores indicate the most overall usefulness of the named herb (for humans). I would say that I pretty much agree with the top ten, except that for cattle I would substitute in ginseng (*Panax ginseng*) instead of gingko, peppermint (*Mentha piperita*) instead of stinging nettle, and move peppermint up the list.

Remember, let your food be your medicine, and as such, get those cows out on the grass as much as possible to enjoy your farm's agroecology.

Garlic	65
Ginger	61
Licorice	54
Echinacea	37
Red Pepper	36
Willow	36
Gingko	33
Evening primrose	27
Stinging nettle	24
Goldenseal	22
Peppermint	19
Pineapple	19
Teatree	16
Camomile	15
Eucalyptus	15
Lemonbalm	14
Rosemary	14
Calendula	13
Purslane	13
Aloe	12
Bilberry	12
Cardamom	12
Honeysuckle	12
Plantain	12
St. John's Wort	12
Chasteberry	11
Dong Quai	11
Pigweed	11
Turmeric	11
Carrot	10
Celery	10
Dandelion	10

Inside the Medicine Bag

I don't usually mention the products that I carry for organic farms, but the other day I was surprised by a farmer when he had no idea about certain treatments I commonly use. These medicines are used within a valid veterinary client-patient relationship (VCPR), which means that a veterinarian has knowledge of the animals in the herd, has been on the farm recently and is available for follow-up, or there is a clinic that is available for follow-up. Here's the list:

Phyto-Mast is a botanical multipurpose antiseptic available in aseptic, easy-to-use tubes with alcohol pads. It is intended to be used as an antiseptic irrigation. Its uses include milk quality, udder rot, pinkeye and digestive upsets. Phyto-Mast may also be considered for cows that have milk quality concerns at dry off. This product is not intended for *Staphylococcus aureus* or coliform infections. The ingredients of Phyto-Mast are essential oil of thyme, licorice, wintergreen, angelica, and vitamin A, D, and E in olive oil.

Get Well is a liquid tincture of plants that have well-known antibacterial properties to enhance health. Get Well is normally used an oral treatment, but I do give it IV as a loading dose when called out for a case (I add it to a carrier such as dextrose or physiologic saline). An oral dose of Get Well is 5cc per calf and 20cc per cow given three times daily. When administered with other IV fluids, a 90cc dose is given. A repeat IV using 60cc in a bottle of dextrose can be given daily as needed.

Heat Seek is a combination of botanicals for reproductive health. It is a botanical blend of herbs that seems to enhance the visually observable signs of heat (estrus). This is for use in animals that are in normal body condition (not skinny/negative energy balance), have a corpus luteum on the ovary, and have not shown visible heats for a long time.

Eat Well is a liquid tincture of plants known to stimulate appetite and the gut. It is purely for indigestion and lack of appetite *with normal temperature (no fever)*. Indications would be mild bloat, constipation, impacted rumen, or potential displaced abomasum. It is an old horse colic remedy as well and works great for that purpose. Eat Well can be given at the rate of 15cc–20cc per adult cow (or horse) or occasionally at 5cc intravenously with a diluent such as dextrose or physiologic saline. Given after IV calcium, this has been shown to help very well.

Ferro is a liquid from water percolated through earth which is high in fulvic acid, iron, sulfur, and almost all the elements on the periodic table. It is especially good at helping animals with diarrhea caused by internal parasites as it constipates them quickly and stops the dehydration. With its high level of iron, Ferro also helps build up the bloodstream in depleted animals. It is given orally. Calves should get 5cc–10cc daily in their milk or mixed with molasses as it is very bitter. Yearlings should get 20cc daily. The duration of treatment is usually seven to ten days. On one farm I took manure samples from the calves infested with giardia. After the treatment, only two of the fifteen or so calves tested had slight amounts of giardia, and they all looked really great compared to pretreatment. Giardia is related to coccidia and cryptosporidia. I normally recommend Ferro for typical stomach worm problems due to strongyle-type worms.

With the above ready in the medicine cabinet, you will be prepared for many situations that can befall organic dairy cows and calves.

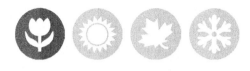

CHAPTER 6

Pasture Bloat, Rumen Acidosis, and Other Pasture Problems

Pasture season is on in full swing. Lush green paddocks and cows wanting to only eat the fresh pasture: a new season of growth is upon us! While you enjoy the season, you may want to keep in mind some problems that can occur with cows out on pasture. What? Cows on pasture can have problems? Well, believe it or not, yes. Pasture bloat, digestive upset, rumen acidosis, and hoof problems are sometimes encountered.

Pasture Bloat

First let's talk about pasture bloat. Pasture bloat occurs when animals are put into really lush legume or legume-grass-mix paddocks for a few days in a row without being offered enough effective fiber or dry hay beforehand, especially in early spring and autumn. It's worse when a frost occurs and the animals are put out to pasture with not a care about frosted forage; you *must* wait two hours until the frost is off before putting animals onto legume pasture. For some reason, bloat itself is only caused by legumes (clovers and alfalfa) as they slowly but surely create millions of tiny bubbles that accumulate over a few days' time. Eventually, they build up to a point where the rumen expands beyond its capacity and the rumen entrance and exit constricts, cutting off the animal's throat, not allowing normal belching/burping of gases that build up within the rumen. This is when the cow rapidly bloats (as seen with a big bulge on their left side), begins to violently kick at her belly because of the extreme pain, can no longer stand, drops down, and can die in short order. Prior to obvious distress, which usually shows on day four or five, a bunch of cows will start to look "fuller"—the animals will appear equally distended on their sides—but will not show any distress. If you put this kind of cow back out on clover or alfalfa pasture another day, she will suffer from pasture bloat. Pasture bloat is entirely

Free-Gas Bloat

Another kind of bloat is free-gas bloat, not associated with grazing, may occur in a single animal (not a whole bunch) and is due to failure to eructate (burp and belch). This can happen any time of year. Usually it is an aftereffect of hardware disease. An animal may bloat on and off for a few days. This condition is a large gas cap in the upper part of the rumen. Passing a tube into the rumen and moving the tube slightly about will usually find the free gas as it will rapidly come out the end of the tube you are holding. Also giving one quart to one half-gallon of either olive oil or mineral oil afterward with one teaspoon of peppermint oil and walking the cow is generally effective. In addition, giving six tablespoons of baking soda (bicarb) in water is good. A calcium bottle IV will also help get the rumen moving, especially if the cow is older and has been milking well. If you use homeopathic remedies, Carbo Veg is a good remedy for an animal with free gas bloat that is cold and near collapse. Colocynthus is a remedy for colic (perhaps due to gas) when an animal looks back to its flank on the bloated side.

preventable, yet every year at this time some herds will lose a cow (or cows) to this problem.

Prevention

Even with proper management, a good farmer may still lose an animal to this kind of bloat each season. When a whole bunch of cows show this problem a few times in a season, it is an indication of a real nutritional problem that needs to be fixed. Usually pasture bloat occurs on the cooler ends of the pasture season, but it can occur at any time. Prevention centers on correct feeding practices. Realize that just because there is lush pasture doesn't mean that nothing else should be fed. Also keep in mind that although grass is a ruminant's natural feed, any sudden feed changes (and especially to extremes) will harm the rumen bugs, which must adapt over a few days to a week's time (different bugs exist at different pH in the rumen, and the correct bugs need time to build up).

The key factor for preventing bloat is to feed cows effective fiber (dry hay) a half-hour before sending them out to gorge on the same lush legume stands again and again for days on end. Use long-stem hay, not the "candy" hay from out west (western alfalfa hay has excellent relative feed value but not as much effective fiber as grass hay). Baleage and haylage will not substitute for actual dry hay because they are already partially digested due to the fermentation process. Using them is better than nothing, but keep in mind they tend to be high in soluble protein themselves, just like pasture.

Homeopathically, give colchicum or colocynthus to a bloated cow if it's still early and the cows just seem a little fuller than normal. Use colchicum if cow doesn't eat, is straining, and doesn't want to move; use colocynthus if she'll move and looks back at her flank. Carbo Veg is a good general homeopathic remedy for any bloating and excessive gassiness in the gut. Give ten pellets or spray the nose every ten to fifteen minutes as needed. Always keep a bloated animal moving about; never put her into a stall to stay tied in. They have a better chance to expel the gas if moving around.

Probably the best thing to do is to alternate through grassy pastures or grassy legume pastures, just not eating straight legume for many days on end. This is when "tall grazing" would make a lot of sense, though early in the season nothing is really tall yet. As far as grasses go, orchard grass is great, but remember that if orchard grass heads out even once in a season, any regrowth will have a different and worse taste to the grazing animals. That's just the biology of orchard grass.

Treatment

Treatment for pasture bloat is rather simple, if you are in time. Give one pint of either vegetable oil (olive oil is best) or mineral oil orally and walk the animal around. Repeat in ten to fifteen minutes if the cow is no better. You can add one teaspoon of peppermint oil into the vegetable/mineral oil to give it flavor so the animal doesn't inhale the liquid into the windpipe. Peppermint has also been shown to help reduce gas in the digestive tract. It is a bit slower acting, but it will do the job. The above treatment has worked nearly all the time for bloat if animals are not yet down. The peppermint and mineral oil are okay for organic. Fortunately, poloxalene (Therabloat) is allowed for emergency use in organics without having to permanently remove the animal from the herd. This treatment is readily effective and will reverse bloat within about two to three minutes. Most people don't keep poloxalene on hand but will have olive oil or mineral oil nearby.

THE KEY FACTOR FOR PREVENTING BLOAT is to feed cows effective fiber (dry hay) a half-hour before sending them out to gorge on the same lush legume stands again and again for days on end.

If a severely bloated cow is down, it is too late for oral oils. In pasture bloat, due to the zillions of tiny bubbles, passing a stomach tube will not relieve the tight rumen. If the animal is down, it is critical to quickly stab the rumen to help expel the excessive rumen pressure that is choking off the animal internally. By standing behind the cow, your left side is her left side and that is the side to stab—generally where the biggest part of the bulge is, just below the short ribs and behind the big ribs. (Do *not* stab the right side of the abdomen—this will cause all sorts of problems since you will be stabbing the intestinal area.) While having to stab a cow is not a fun thought, it is necessary to save its life if the animal is down. Use a short, sturdy knife the length of your fist. Make a quick thrust in, *and then turn your hand ninety degrees to open up the slit you just created.* A small volcanic eruption with lots of tiny bubbles will burst forth, and relief will be immediate. Amazingly, these stab wounds don't usually cause too much of a problem afterward. Though they certainly can lead to peritonitis (generalized belly infection), fresh forage seems to cause much less problems (as opposed to only fermented feeds during the non-grazing season). I can't explain it, but I have seen surprisingly good results from stabs to cows severely bloated from pasture. This procedure should have to be done only once in a couple of years' time. If it happens more frequently, ask yourself how you can prevent bloat rather than resorting to stabbing your cows.

Digestive Problems

Above all, radically changing the diet of the herd by putting them all out onto lush growing pasture can cause digestive upsets. Try putting cows on grass for only a few hours a day early in the season while still feeding the dry hay and/or long leaf baleage in the barn. Moving cows quickly through fields (flash grazing) at this point will keep them from trampling young growth too much. Keep them in a paddock for an hour or two and move on. This mimics the constant movements of wild ruminants like the American bison, so it is a very natural thing for the cows to move along. Transition your cows to twelve-hour grazing by going from two to three hours per day in pleasant afternoons to both morning and afternoon grazing over a week's time. It's understandable that people want to get their cows out of the barn, but try to do it in a way that doesn't hamper the early growth of your pastures; otherwise you might be shooting yourself in the foot.

Once pasture is in full gear, we often notice cows with pipe-stream "pasture" manure. What does this mean? Simply put: excessive rumen-degradable protein (soluble protein). Fast-growing grass in the vegetative state is chock-full of protein, but way too much for a cow's rumen to handle and remain healthy. All that protein from the pasture creates ammonia as it's broken down. That ammonia can seep through the rumen walls. The cow's system takes care of it by sending it to the liver, which converts the ammonia to urea (this process was previously covered in chapter 7). This urea enters the bloodstream and is called blood urea nitrogen (BUN). BUN is mostly turned into urine and excreted, but it also freely moves into the udder and creates milk urea nitrogen (MUN). This whole process is the cow's way of getting rid of too much protein, but transforming the excessive ammonia costs the cow biological energy and lowers milk production, and is part of the reason why we often see cows on prime pasture getting lean. But we can reduce this excessive drain on their system in two simple ways: first by making sure that there is enough *energy* for them to balance out the excessive protein being taken in, and second by slowing down the rate of passage through the rumen by feeding *effective fiber*. The best effective fiber to slow down digestion is dry hay, but cows tend to dislike the dried feeds when they have lush green salad to enjoy in the springtime. They will eat it, though, if you pour or spray diluted molasses on it (or soak a bale with molasses a few hours before feeding it), and the molasses will provide energy to the rumen as well. And while many farmers that are into grazing do not like the thought of corn silage (even though it's a grass itself), corn silage actually complements grazing well because it provides energy and fiber—and cows still like it even when on pasture. Regardless, balancing the intake of protein, fiber, and energy are primary factors for proper nutrition for your cows' sake.

Grass Tetany

What about grass tetany? Grass tetany is low blood levels of magnesium. Grass tetany occurs when there is lush growth of pasture; however, it can be any kind of pasture (not just bloat-causing legumes);

grass tetany is actually more likely on grass stands. It will more quickly affect a fresh cow that has more metabolic needs than a later lactation cow. Its symptoms are somewhat like milk fever, and in actuality they easily could occur together. The main symptoms include stiffness in a leg or body side (unlike milk fever where muscles are weak and lax). The cow will almost fall over but usually immediately right herself, but after this goes on a while she will lie down. However, cows are very uncomfortable when lying down because the muscles in certain areas will become stiff. They can also then all of a sudden get up with normal strength (unlike a milk fever), and this back-and-forth can go on for a while. They will act a bit more agitated than usual (similar to early milk fever) and stay that way (whereas with milk fever they will become depressed and dull). A recent history of eating early pasture growth will aid in the diagnosis and its subsequent proper treatment.

Treatment consists of correcting the metabolic disturbance by giving magnesium, either orally in the form of large capsules of Epsom salts (magnesium sulfate) or six to ten large "pink pills" (magnesium oxide), or by giving intravenous CMPK (calcium, magnesium, phosphorus and potassium). However, it can be darn difficult to hit a vein properly in a cow that wants to keep shifting around when it is standing while it also partially attempts to lay down. Just wait until it is down, then put a halter on her and tie the halter to a non-mobile post. Don't tie it back to her leg like in milk fever because of the strength she can use to try to get free (and mess up your IV needle position). Give the bottle at no higher than her backbone (since it has calcium in it). If it is an older cow, continue into a second bottle, and if you have a stethoscope handy listen to the heart to make sure it is beating regularly (it may be at a quicker rate, but it should be beating totally regularly) while you give the entire second bottle. By the end, the cow should be noticeably calmer than prior to treatment. Regular 23 percent calcium IV will *not* work; the treatment *must* have magnesium in it. Follow-up treatment includes administering the "pink pills" or Epsom salt.

Cows left untreated and found down and unable to rise will often show more severe neurologic symptoms, such as paddling the ground area near them, and will have a staring expression. They then may con-

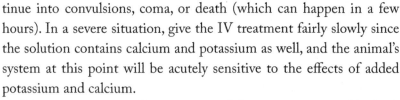

tinue into convulsions, coma, or death (which can happen in a few hours). In a severe situation, give the IV treatment fairly slowly since the solution contains calcium and potassium as well, and the animal's system at this point will be acutely sensitive to the effects of added potassium and calcium.

Grass tetany is caused by pastures with low magnesium and/or high potassium. Magnesium absorption is reduced when the concentration of ammonia in the rumen is high (as with lush pasture of any sort). The combination of low-magnesium pastures and rapid growth leads to this condition. Although rare, it may be seen during spring.

Rumen Acidosis

Every spring I usually get at least a few calls from alarmed farmers that cows on lush pasture are suffering from, believe it or not, *rumen acidosis*. Oftentimes graziers will reflexively say that rumen acidosis only occurs on conventional confinement farms, due to the practice of feeding large amounts of grain and insufficient fiber to push for really high milk production. While rumen acidosis is more commonly seen any time of year on farms that feed a combination of high amounts of corn silage, high-moisture corn, and grain supplements fed out as a TMR, believe it or not it can also hit grazing cows that milk more moderate levels of grain feeding. Why?

First, let's look at what rumen acidosis is. Normal healthy rumen pH should be about 6.8. The pH tells you how much acid is in a system, whether you're measuring the soil that your crops grow in, your well water, or a cow's rumen. As the system becomes more acidic, the pH number goes towards zero. The pH is also a "log" number, which means that a one point drop from 6.0 to 5.0 indicates that there is now ten times more acid in the system. The population of microbes in the rumen is highly varied, and each type of bug is sensitive to a certain range of pH. Some of the digestion products the rumen creates are dependent on the general rumen ecology, which is affected by the pH. When all the bugs are "happy," there will be a lot of production of acetic and propionic acid, with some butyric acid. These are volatile fatty acids that can migrate through the rumen wall and enter the cow's

Watching for Rumen Health

We all know that grazing is more of an art than a science, but just because cows are on green grass it doesn't necessarily mean that their rumens are happy and healthy. Perhaps one of the best and easiest ways to watch rumen health is to let your cows tell you how they are doing. Do they chew *at least sixty chews per cud* that they bring up? It's easy to do—simply count the chews they chew of a cud right after they bring it up. Do it with a bunch of cows. *If chewing less than fifty chews per cud, they are lacking fiber for the rumen mat.* That is actually vital biological information to know. Also, are at least 60 percent of the cows chewing cud an hour after eating? What does the manure look like? With good digestive health, manure should not shoot out of cows like water from a hose but instead should "set up." It also shouldn't have any whole grain in it. That's money going right through your cows without any benefit to you. Truly, feeding stored forage can beautifully balance out lush, green grass quite nicely. By taking some simple steps, you can make sure that your cows are healthy and happy when out on pasture this season.

general system to help build certain milk components (acetic acid, for example, which generally helps build butterfat). When the rumen pH drops much below 6.0, the normal rumen bugs are unhappy and die off, especially if the pH remains too low for too long and then lactic acid–loving bacteria will predominate. Rumen acidosis is then happening, burning the walls of the rumen.

The pH, being a reflection of the amount of acid present, can be changed very easily by the cow's intake of different feed ingredients. To keep the rumen bugs happy, cows chew cud. Chewing cud creates saliva, which has bicarbonate in it and opposes acid. Therefore, the more the cows chew cud, the more saliva they produce, and this saliva when swallowed with the cud maintains a rumen pH between 6.0 and 7.0, keeping the important microbes happy. What makes cows chew cud? Fiber. The best fiber for cud chewing is dry hay. You can never have enough dry hay on a dairy farm. Dry hay is nearly medicinal feed for cows. Fresh grasses and legumes from pasture also provide a lot of material for cud chewing, but sometimes the effective fiber is not as great. We easily see this when cows shoot "pasture manure" across the walkways at this time of the season.

What is almost the opposite of healthy fiber? Grain. The purpose of grain is primarily to provide energy for cows to make lots of milk. Grain feeding tends to favor propionic acid–producing bugs. Propionic acid is the volatile acid that contributes to higher levels of milk production. In the wild, ruminants do eat grain by way of seed heads on grasses and the like. So while grain is not entirely foreign to a cow's system, giving too much hammers the system in a terrible way. As grain ferments in the rumen, it produces lactic acid, which will drop the rumen pH lower and lower unless offset by sufficient fiber intake. The whole science of ruminant nutrition essentially boils down to balancing the amount of fiber and grain going into the rumen to keep the bugs happy and to produce milk. How this is accomplished definitely affects cow health.

The health of a cow (or any ruminant) depends on a healthy rumen. A ruminant by definition chews cud. The amount of cud chewing, especially *chews per cud*, is a quick way to evaluate the health of a cow's rumen. A cow should chew anywhere from fifty to seventy chews *per cud* that is brought up. This is easy to watch and fun to do. If there are less than fifty chews per cud on a significant number of animals, their diet is lacking in fiber. If grain is coming through in the manure or the manure is not consistent between herd animals, this will confirm rumen acidosis.

With all this in mind, perhaps you can see how rumen acidosis can occur *with grazing herds*. In grazing herds that feed grain (which most do to some extent), there must be adequate effective fiber going into the rumen so the cow chews cud as much as possible to maximize saliva production with its bicarbonate. I have seen grazing herds on lush spring grass that get rumen acidosis by "slug feeding" grain twice a day (even as little as six pounds per feeding) at milking times and not consuming dry hay but only baleage, or worse, haylage (short chop). *Always* feed hay before grain. *Never* feed grain to cows straight after pasture—it's way too much highly fermentable starch for the rumen to handle after other rapidly fermentable sugars from pasture are already in the rumen. Always put some kind of forage out first; then feed the grain.

Typical signs of rumen acidosis include decreased or no cud chewing, loose or diarrhea manure, becoming skinny, decreased milk, and possibly teeth grinding. The treatment is rather simple: long-stem dry hay, free-choice or force-fed baking soda (sodium bicarbonate), and rumen probiotics to repopulate the rumen with "good bugs." This treatment will be needed for a few days until manure stabilizes and appetite improves. If a cow is truly acidotic, she will eagerly eat dry hay to the exclusion of other feeds. Always try to feed the most nutrient-dense forages to cows to keep the rumen healthy and maintain good body condition. At least 60 percent of resting cows should be chewing cud at any time and each cud ideally chewed sixty times.

Hoof Problems for Cows on Pasture

Unfortunately, the consequences of rumen acidosis are many, but an obvious one is on the hooves. With the permeability of the rumen walls increased due to the biochemical burning of the walls by the acidosis, pathogenic toxins can escape into the animal's circulation. The circulation down to the hoof area is very complex and delicate, and suffice it to say that interference with normal circulation can cause an upset in the integrity and health of the hoof-hairline junction. With any weakness created, the bacteria presumed to cause strawberry heel have a better chance of taking hold in that area (especially when cows stand around in mud and muck) and create the characteristic lesion. The sickness also alters the the general growth of the hoof, and anytime that happens other problems can take advantage of the weakened hoof structure. It is interesting to see in some herds that the hooves of all the cows have a line on them (parallel to the hoof-hairline junction)—this is diagnostic of rumen acidosis having occurred or at a minimum, a significant digestive upset of some kind.

> I believe that the give and take of the natural earth underneath the animals as they walk on pasture helps prevent sole ulcers even if the conditions for rumen acidosis are present.

However, the consequences of rumen acidosis, particularly on hoof health, don't seem to be as terrible in grazing herds as on those always kept inside on concrete barnyards. I believe that the give and take of the natural earth underneath the animals as they walk on pasture helps prevent sole ulcers even if the conditions for rumen acidosis are present. This theory has been borne out by seeing a few outbreaks of a bunch of cows getting into grain and becoming very ill but having no long-term lameness issues due to sole ulcers.

In chronic, low-grade rumen acidosis (also called subacute rumen acidosis or SARA), sole ulcers will develop on the bottom of the hoof. These are always on the bottom, about a third of the way forward from the back heel and two-thirds back from the toe tip. These are classic signs of rumen acidosis. On grazing herds that I know who get a hoof trimmer in, sole ulcers are almost never noted.

Lameness not due to acute acidosis or chronic acidosis is another problem at this time of year. As the cows walk on laneways to pasture, they undoubtedly have a higher potential to suffer from hoof punctures and sprains. Hoof puncture potential is compounded by walking lanes that have many stones in them (on the surface or submerged in muddy areas), by cows standing in creeks with unseen stones on the bottom, or simply standing in muck and soupy areas.

Hoof problems decrease the enjoyment of cows out on pasture. Abscesses occur when stones puncture the bottom of hooves that are already soft from standing in manure or wet areas. Abscesses also occur when the ground is hard and dry—when there is no "give"—and the hoof gets punctured when full weight is applied to it during walking. White-colored hooves, regardless of animal species, tend to be softer and more prone to problems than black-colored hooves because of their different biochemical make-up. While black hooves tend to be more resistant to problems, they are much harder to work on with hoof knives and nippers since they are harder and more brittle.

Although foot rot is technically contagious like hairy heel wart is, it seems to mainly occur to animals that have stepped on something sharp between the two toes. A swelling can quickly develop above the hoof-hairline junction, indicating an infected joint. For a long time I thought that such a condition would require antibiotics but I have found that using a mix of sugar and povidone iodine (Betadine) works fantastically. People from around the world have told me they agree. Take half a cup granular sugar and add twenty milliliters of povidone iodine and mix well to make a thick blob. This mix makes for three treatments. Apply to cotton and wrap with a hoof wrap so the toes are spread apart. In three days, take off the bandage and a dead core of material will drop out (if not, pull it out). Then cleanse and rewrap with another blob of sugar-povidone iodine on cotton and wrap again. The swelling above the hoof-hairline junction tends to come out quickly. You can take off the second wrap three days later. Repeat one time if needed.

Installing a box with a dry hydrated lime that the cows must walk through is a nice antiseptic and preventative for contagious problems. It is less messy than the copper sulfate baths and will not quickly max out your soil's copper levels. Perhaps adding in some dry copper sulfate powder to the hydrated lime would be better yet.

While I previous discussed ketosis (lack of energy) and how to prevent it, you also need to be aware that too much energy *coupled with a lack of fiber* can severely impact cows in a very bad way. It all comes down to a balanced approach to feeding and not being too extreme in one direction or the other. Each and every grazier really should be connected with a nutritionist, one who is truly interested in proper grazing and basing the ration on the growing grass as the primary ingredient. Do not try to work with a nutritionist that simply pays lip service to grazing to keep your business. It is usually fairly obvious who truly likes to work with grazing herds and who doesn't.

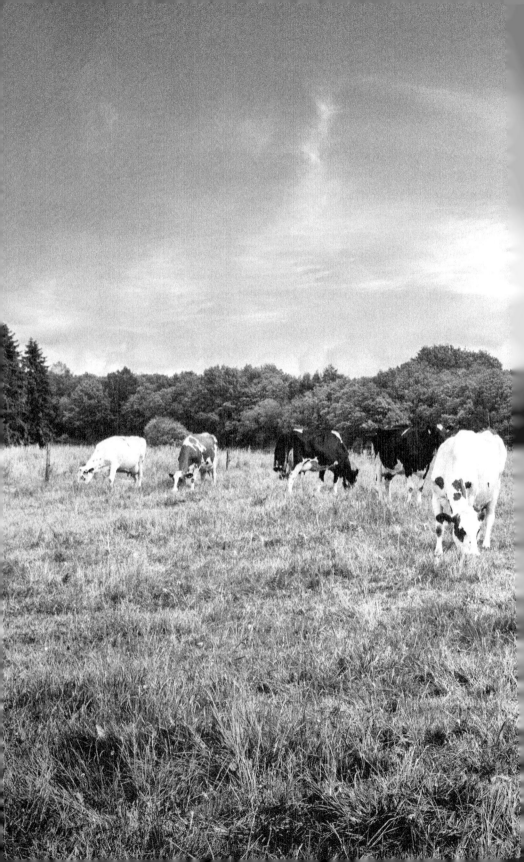

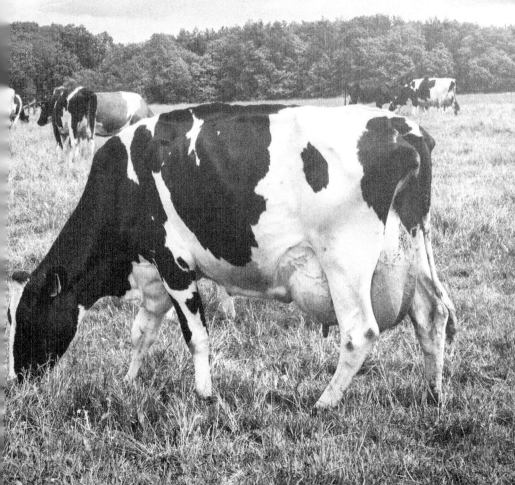

PART II

Summer

CHAPTER 7

Parasites

Spring and summer are here, the grass is finally growing, and the scent of flowers is in the air. Everything is growing: pastures, calves—and parasites. Parasites love warmth and humidity. Unless you're in a drought-stricken area and *extremely* dry, the warm, humid summer weather helps parasites multiply in a very short amount of time. Parasites are those creatures that serve no real purpose but to live for themselves at the expense of other living beings. Parasites can be internal or external. Important internal livestock parasites include stomach worms and coccidia. There are many more, but those two probably cause the most problems to most organic dairy farmers. External parasites bring to mind flies, lice, and mange. (By the way, ringworm is not a parasite but a fungus that grows on the outermost layer of skin.) Flies torment animals during the warm season while the effects of lice and mange tend to be seen during the indoor housing times of colder season.

I really think that parasitism, whether internal or external, is truly the weak link in the chain of organic livestock health and growth. I say this after being in practice for many years now, seeing untold numbers of cases of parasitized animals. I see crummy-looking calves out on pasture during the summer, especially later summer—"naturally raised," certified organic, *and* conventional raised. Parasites (of any kind) will always be present wherever there is a high animal density in a contained area. Only the free-roaming bison on the American Plains could constantly move ahead and not encounter heavy pressure of internal parasites. However, a major way to reduce that pressure while keeping your animals healthier within your farm's boundaries is to feed them really well so they have the wherewithal to fend off inevitable parasite challenges. So the overall strategy is to figure out how to minimize the "feast" (your animals) for the parasites, hopefully without chemical methods to which the quickly reproducing parasites will become resistant in short order.

Causes of Infection

If you're pasturing animals in the same areas year after year, you've got to realize that there will be parasites waiting for each group as they arrive since many parasite eggs can survive over winter in the soil waiting for warm and moist conditions to return. Pastures look really nice early on, but those stomach worm larvae are invisible to our eyes and are rapidly multiplying and loading the animals that are out there eating the forages. Right now, unless your paddocks are scorched dry, parasites are thriving and sending millions of eggs out onto pasture as your herd animals drop their manure on the ground. The eggs hatch in a few hours, the larvae of the stomach worms then crawl up the blades of nearby grass, hoping to be eaten by animals as they graze, then start their life again in the host, sucking blood from the stomach walls. This is basic biology of the strongyle class of internal worms—which affects not only cattle, but sheep, goats, pigs, horses, and many other mammals—and there's no getting around it completely.

Parasites always take advantage of the fact that animals on farms are enclosed in the same spot due to perimeter fencing or indoor stalls and cannot get away from them. Free-roaming cattle on the original prairie probably had a low level of parasitism with which they could live in balance. Parasites generally thrive under these conditions: high animal density, animals kept in the same areas continuously, nutritionally deprived animals, poor pasture management, and poor premises management. Coccidia are usually found in animals indoors in pens that are being continually used. Coccidia problems are not usually seen when animals are on pasture. On the other hand, stomach worms are usually found in animals on pasture (and not when continuously inside), especially at peak and late season when the parasite population has multiplied many times. This buildup is due to cattle reinfecting the pastures in the warm, humid months with fresh manure carrying worm eggs ready to hatch and be eaten again with pasture grass. It is critical to never have young stock follow older stock—young stock immune systems are not capable of withstanding parasitism like mature adult cattle can. And, importantly, Johne's disease can also be passed to younger animals following older animals on pasture. It is very rare that adult cows need any kind of wormer at all, unless you want to increase milk production a few pounds per day. Adult cows can and do carry stomach worms but they do not become infested; check some manure samples and you'll see. However, young stock can get hammered by parasites. Interestingly, a very low level of parasites will probably create a stronger animal than one that is routinely dewormed. Only by checking manure samples can the level of infection be known.

Also contributing to parasitism is the harmful practice of not feeding hay to pre-weaned calves. Why is this harmful? In the search to satisfy their instinctual need for fiber, calves will eat bedding, which will likely have parasites on it. Just watch some calves for a while that do not get any hay fed to them—they will nibble the ground for fibrous material, guaranteed. Additionally, the developing rumen (which causes the instinct to want fiber) is not just a "sponge" that absorbs and passes on volatile fatty acids (supplied most quickly by grain); it is also a muscular organ that turns over every minute or two. The muscles develop more strongly with hay in the diet. Ever see bloating pre-weaned calves? Their diet is usually milk replacer and grain—no hay until after weaning.

In organic agriculture, due in part to the requirement that animals six months and older must get a minimum of 30 percent dry matter from pasture over the grazing season, it is only a matter of time before the young stock, which are not immunologically mature against stomach worms, will become infested if pasture management is not top-notch. A big part of pasture management is proper feeding to ensure excellent energy intake while on pasture, such as from high-energy forages or some grain. The immune system depends heavily on proper daily energy intake.

I think a good goal is to raise calves that do have *some* challenge from stomach worm larva in the pasture yet are managed and fed well enough that rather than becoming infested, they instead build immunity due to a low-level exposure. This is a kind of a natural vaccine effect. Unfortunately, not many farms seem to be able to achieve this low level of exposure. The result is somewhat stunted calves that likely will freshen a month or two later since they won't reach breeding size as quickly. However, calves that do make it through this tough period of life—usually between four and eleven months of age—start looking *really* nice again by a year old and go on to do fine. Even if they did look crummy due to a significant stomach worm infestation, they will now be strong against pasture stomach worm challenges the rest of their lives.

Signs and Symptoms

Unfortunately, the smaller the land base and higher the animal density, the more likely it is that parasites will infest young stock as similar groups are placed in the same small lots year after year. Animals carrying a burden of internal worms will suffer from lowered immune systems, which can be troublesome if there are sudden changes in weather (cool damp weather will quickly trigger the calves to start coughing). Only on rare occasions have I seen an animal so severely parasitized that they are near dead due to anemia (loss of blood due to parasite action). This will present as an animal that has a swollen-looking jaw (fluid filled), very white mucous membranes (mouth, eye sockets, vulva), and is extremely weak—most likely lying down. Sometimes these young animals will also have ulcers in their mouth.

What do your calves on pasture look like right now? Are they sleek and in good body condition, just like when you weaned them or set them out to pasture? Or do they look a bit more ragged now, perhaps a bit potbellied, their hair dry and reddish-black, not shiny black as it should be? Do they have thin back-leg muscles and dried diarrhea high on their legs and tail? If so, these are classic signs of internal stomach worm infestation.

It would be wise to catch up a few calves and look in their eye sockets to see how pink or pale white the sockets are. In sheep and goats, it is common to use the FAMACHA (Faffa Malan Chart) test, which involves looking at their eye sockets. How white the sockets are, indicating anemia, will indicate when to treat them with a conventional wormer. While the FAMACHA test is technically not valid for calves, looking at their eye sockets will nonetheless reveal the degree of blood loss. Calves just hide it until later in the disease.

Remember, really check your young stock on pasture for signs of internal worm infestation. If they are infested and nothing is done about it, the first batch of damp cold weather will likely bring on pneumonia—and that is not at all desirable. So be mindful: stop and observe your animals and take action as needed now, not later.

Prevention and Treatment

As the summer progresses, remember to address parasite prevention and treatment in young stock from a multipronged approach, which is a logical response because:

1. A variety of approaches for any problem will give a better chance of success.
2. If one pillar of the multipronged approach isn't working, the other factors are still in place.
3. Natural treatments can work well.
4. There will be less chance of resistance developing.

If you are used to giving calves a systemic wormer (like ivermectin or moxidectin) and you replace it with some natural wormer, this would be what is called "input substitution," the opposite of a multipronged approach. What we really need to do is understand the biology of the parasites that like to live in or on cattle and then figure out where to break their life cycle. Only after that can we go on to use a botanical mixture to substitute for the typically used synthetic wormer.

Worms

For internal parasites, we need to address not only when the parasites are in the animal, but also when they are outside the animal in the environment. We need to think about how to make the environment hostile to them. In general, all life does better with moisture. Therefore, we need to dry out the areas where parasites would be happiest. This means splattering out the manure patties in the pasture and/or putting hogs and chickens in the pasture to quickly sift through the manure patties, exposing the patties to the wind and sun and thereby drying them out. We need dung beetles as well. Some wormers, especially ivermectin, are very harmful to dung beetles.

We also need to make sure that the animals are in robust nutritional condition so that their immune systems can handle and tolerate the likely parasite challenge. Weaned calves are usually the hardest hit because they do not have enough body condition when sent out to the pasture to fend for themselves. To get a calf in top body condition (in order to endure the stresses associated with post-weaning), keep them on whole milk for at least three months, then wean slowly over two weeks. If you have high-quality pasture for your young stock, they will grow well without the need for grain. However, if excellent pasture is not provided, you need to feed additional forages and concentrates or those calves will crash and become malnourished, heavily parasitized, anemic, and scour (and some will die). I see this every year on some farms.

This disaster can be avoided by paying extra attention to their nutritional needs and feeding what is needed before it is too late. By keeping nutrition where it should be and by reducing the moisture where parasite larvae live, the need for wormers (of any type) will be significantly reduced. I can confidently say that calves that are well fed do not need wormers. Calves that have been well fed but are on marginal-quality pasture with no clipping/dragging (where worm larvae can build up) and are exposed to an increasing population of worms over the summer season may respond fairly well to natural botanical wormers, which would break the cycle of the parasites within the animal. However, the animals' environment better be cleaned up and better managed if this approach is to work well.

Flies

For external parasites, like flies, we again need to consider areas where moisture builds up, especially areas with big accumulations of moisture-laden manure. Fly populations explode with humid air, heat, thundershower activity, moisture/sweat, and manure on the animals to attract them. Of course we cannot control the weather, but we can determine what kind of environment our animals live in. Do they slop around in "soup" near their feeding area (including round bale feed areas)? Do they lie in areas that are moist and damp? Do they lie under the only tree in the pasture, making a mud hole? Is there such a buildup of bedding in their outdoor superhutch that a slow, steady trickle of fluid is draining away from it? Are the animals forced to plunge their faces down through tall, rank pasture growth to get at the more lush vegetation nearer to the ground, leading the cows to prick their eyes on the taller, less-appetizing plants and causing tearing (moisture)? Tears running from the animals' eyes makes for pinkeye in short order. All these conditions attract flies, in addition to stacked manure that is aging (stacked either on purpose or due to "natural" buildup from not being mucked out regularly).

> **FOR EXTERNAL PARASITES,** like flies, we again need to consider areas where moisture builds up, especially areas with big accumulations of moisture-laden manure.

"Clean and dry" are cardinal terms for the keeping of livestock. While the best efforts to keep animals clean and dry can still be opposed by weather conditions that encourage flies, it is the foundation

Types of Flies

Horn flies are smaller than other kinds of flies and are usually found on the bellies and backs of cows. Horn flies deposit eggs in fresh manure, and they take nine to twelve days to develop into adults. They take ten to twelve blood meals per day and can transmit *Staphylococcus aureus* between animals. Face flies also lay eggs in fresh manure and become adults in fourteen days. Face flies have been found to carry more than thirty bacterial diseases and are the main carriers of the pinkeye bug. Stable flies are found on the lower body and legs of cattle and take about two to three blood meals a day. They prefer aging manure and bedding or round bale feeder areas to deposit their eggs. Cattle bunch up trying to avoid their painful bites. House flies will use a variety of organic materials to lay their eggs, and it takes about seven days for them to become adults.[*]

Wes Watson and Steve Demming, "Managing Parasite Flies in Pasture-based Dairy Systems," presented at the Mid-Atlantic Grazing Conference, July 2012.

for pest prevention, to be put in place before trying "band-aids" to help during problem times.

Methods of reducing the effects of flies include sticky tape, pheromones to attract flies into traps, tunnel ventilation (moves air so flies cannot land and keeps the animals drier), tails on cows to swat flies away, pouring liberal amounts of field lime on the animals to keep the moisture/sweat away, and proper nutrition (as flies seem to be attracted to animals that are sick, have liver problems, etc.). Then, after all these are incorporated, a fly spray like Ecto-Phyte (Agri-Dynamics) will help quite a bit. But do not simply rely on a natural fly spray instead of an organophosphate fly spray. The difference between simple-minded input substitution and a wise, holistic, multipronged approach will become readily apparent.

So how do we treat internal parasite infestations on certified organic farms? Ivermectin, moxidectin and fenbendazole are allowed to be used but only for an emergency after methods acceptable to organic have not succeeded in restoring an animal to health. A ninety-day milk withhold is required if lactating cows are treated. There is some discussion to reduce the ninety days to seven or ten days. Typically in the past I have recommended a synthetic wormer as a one-time treatment—essentially to reset the individual animals infested—and then get the management in place to keep things in prevention mode rather than reaction (treatment) mode.

Fortunately, there are also many plant-based medicines being used around the world against internal parasites. In the chapter I wrote called "Phytotherapy for Dairy Cows" in the book *Veterinary Herbal Medicine*,* I reported on a study that showed birdsfoot trefoil or chickory interplanted into pasture decreased the stomach worm larva burden significantly compared to a straight white clover and rye pasture. This is because of tannins contained in the birdsfoot trefoil and chickory.

What should we treat with later in the grazing season if our young stock looks crummy? Treatments can range from materials that are high in tannins, like black walnut hulls; dewormer mixes that are added to the feed; to Ferro, which has extremely high levels of humates, iron and minerals. One treatment is to give 10cc of Ferro once daily for five days in a row. This course of treatment is highly effective but requires dosing individual animals, which most farmers understandably do not like to do when it comes to a group of heifers outside. Any herbal formulas with ginger, garlic and neem would be helpful to battle internal parasites in the digestive tract. Another option to try would be Neema-Tox or Vermi-Tox from Agri-Dynamics. Vermi-Tox was shown to have positive benefits in clinical trials at Chico State University. In that study, Vermi-Tox and ivermectin gave equally good reduction of fecal egg counts whereas the no-treatment group became much worse. Weaned cattle are dosed at one ounce per

---

* Susan G. Wynne and Barbara Fougère, Veterinary Herbal Medicine (St. Louis, MO: Mosby, 2007).

three hundred to four hundred pounds for three days in a row. Remember, you *can* use a synthetic wormer if your animals are in really bad shape, and you probably should at that point. Bear in mind, however, that ivermectin is totally poisonous to the dung beetle population, those friendly beetles that decompose manure paddies quickly in healthy biological systems.

If a farm is found using a synthetic wormer on a certain age class of animals every year, most certifiers would rightly ask to see what the farm is doing to prevent parasite pressures from developing. By using rotational pasture management so animals get new paddocks every twelve hours and by giving the grazed paddocks a rest in order to regrow. Just as important, dragging pastures to spread out manure will allow quicker drying out of manure to kill the fragile microscopic larva crawling about. The ideal time to drag out manure pies is three days from when the cows are on the paddock, which will not hinder pasture regrowth and more importantly will allow the dung beetles to do their incredibly important work, drilling manure into channels they create in the soil. This timing also allows time for horn flies and face flies to lay their eggs, so eggs will be hatched and the fragile young larva can also be killed by spreading out the manure pies and quickly drying out the living areas of internal parasites and developing flies.

Conventional farms can put an ear tag into an animal that gives a slow release insecticide to the animal's system to kill flies when they bite the animal. The manure from such an animal will also kill flies or fly larvae that feed on the manure (both good and bad bugs are killed). Insecticide ear tags as well as regular fly sprays and the blue "sprinkles" are prohibited for use on organic farms. In most years, a combination, multi-prong approach to fly control on organic farms can be fairly effective. The following are usual methods of controlling flies—and remember that it is a *combination* of these approaches that works best. You are fooling yourself if you think that using only one or two approaches will work. The list includes: sticky paper in the barns, pheromone fly traps, wasp predators routinely placed in strategic areas, botanical fly sprays applied daily, hanging barrel feeders with salt in the pasture with solar-powered sprayers, electric zappers that animals walk through and of course clean, dry cows (since flies are attracted to moisture) and tunnel ventilation.

When farmers apply concepts of biology, chronic problems like flies can be managed better. Take for instance that flies like warm, humid conditions and flies don't like wind. How many times are you bothered by flies on a windy day? Applying this basic concept to farms would indicate that air flow in the barn would mean dramatically less fly problems. Lo and behold, go into a barn that has tunnel ventilation and you will experience few if any flies. It certainly need not be tunnel ventilation, but something about tunnel ventilation simply works extremely well against flies.

You have probably heard by now of the Spalding Cow-Vac, a machine that generates high-velocity wind in a walk-through chamber. It also has a vacuum aspect that sucks the flies that have been blown off the cows into a large jar. Without a doubt this is the best way to reduce the amount of flies tormenting your cows as well as eliminating them from the breeding population, thereby lowering fly numbers throughout the fly season. The Spalding Cow-Vac is now commercially available (see your trade magazines). It was developed at North Carolina State University.

While I will always promote a multipronged approach to solving problems, if there was ever a "one-stop shopping" method of dealing with flies, the wind/vacuum chamber is it. While other methods like sticky tape catch random flies and parasitic wasps will help reduce the number of flies that become adults, the fly-vac basically wipes out large numbers quickly—right off the cows—which will make your cows more comfortable, allowing them to graze better. The fly-vac may well be the single best invention yet for non-chemical fly control.

As the seasons change, young animals carrying parasite burdens are especially susceptible to damp, chilly air, especially if brought indoors once the pasture season is over. Never, ever bring young stock back inside to a building that shares air with older animals. A rule of thumb is that once an animal leaves the main barn where it was housed as a youngster, always raise it outdoors (with proper shelter) and bring it back into the main adult barn only when it is ready to join the milking string. Too many times I have been called to see sick and coughing parasitized animals that were brought back into the barn in October or November when the weather got bad. Major mistake. By feeding animals well and keeping them outdoors in managed pastures and shelters, your young stock will grow up to become healthy, productive members of your dairy herd.

In summary, make sure you clip your pastures to splatter out manure patties to expose the worm larvae to the drying effects of sun and wind. This will also give uniform regrowth. Also keep animals off a paddock three weeks before putting them back on, as worm larvae need to be ingested by then to complete their life cycle inside the animal. And *never* have young stock follow adults through paddocks, as adults can live in balance with the worms they shed but *will* infect young stock. Immunity to worms usually starts becoming effective at about twelve months of age.

CHAPTER 8

Pinkeye

To keep with seasonal topics, this chapter is dedicated to that pesky condition pinkeye. It's interesting how people often will play the odds, hoping that it won't be a bad pinkeye year. It is nearly impossible to predict how bad a given year will be; however, every year various herds will experience pinkeye problems. In my home area in southeastern Pennsylvania, pinkeye tends to start showing up, on average, in early July and runs through mid September. It corresponds to a buildup of continual hot, humid air—especially with summer thunderstorm activity. Incidence is also related to fly pressures due to manure buildup in various areas of the livestock operation.

Pinkeye is an infection of the outer layer of the eye. The infectious germ that causes it, *Moraxella bovis*, is a bacteria carried from animal to animal mainly by flies. Anything that attracts flies to animals will increase the chance of pinkeye as well as other fly-associated problems, i.e. mastitis in lactating cows, dry cows, and young immature heifers. Pinkeye is an infection sets up an intensely painful condition in the affected animal. Fortunately animals usually only have one affected eye, but some very unlucky animals will have both eyes affected and be blind for a few weeks. The first sign of infection is when an animal looks "weepy and sleepy" and has a watery discharge from the eye, usually running down its jaw. This will attract more flies. Then they will squint their eye shut due to intense pain, which lasts for many days. The eye then opens again but looks all white and aggravated, temporarily blind, and may end up ulcerating, possibly becoming permanently blind.

Pinkeye is the classic case of a combination of factors giving rise to a pesky but not fatal disease. This infection is a good example of the term "holistic management" and whether it can be seen working in practice or not (By "holistic" I mean using every available means possible to combat infection or disease). The three underlying factors that cause pinkeye are stress, nutrition, and environment. If these are out of balance, then the flies that carry the pinkeye germ will start to do damage. It is rare, in my experience, that pinkeye hits animals when all three factors are in balance, but it can happen if there is an unusually potent strain of pinkeye on the farm.

The animals most likely to contract pinkeye are weanlings and fresh cows. Why these two groups? Mainly because they are under the most stress, and their immune system is not at peak strength. For fresh cows, the stress upon their system is due to calving and the major internal changes taking place, which lowers their immune response capability. Mostly, however, it's the younger animals that get pinkeye—especially those born in late winter or early spring, weaned by June or July, and put outside on the same paddock used every year by that age group of animal. Parasites, in the form of bloodsucking stomach worm larvae, are waiting on the tips of grass blades, wanting to be ingested so they can reproduce inside the animal. Their presence will draw down the immune system of the host animal, and many bad things can then happen, pinkeye being just one of them. Weanlings, especially those already weaned for one to four months when the flies first make their appearance, are also stressed from the nutritional change from a rich milk diet to usually the poorest feed on the farm. Environmental factors behind pinkeye for both weanlings and other animals include unclipped pastures, which will cause animals to push their faces down through dry, mature growth to get to the lush growth underneath. They will likely poke their eyes upon the rank upper growth, causing their eyes to water and attract flies and the variety of germs they carry.

Animals in good body condition with the correct balance of protein, energy, and minerals in their ration will likely be able to mount an immune response to the bacteria that flies carry. Adding extra vitamin A and iodine can help eye health. The iodine can be from kelp or iodine tincture added to the water trough. I've seen pinkeye on both conventional and organic farms, but there have been some years that I've had more farms with no pinkeye at all, both conventional and organic, even though it'd been a really terrible fly year due to all the moisture and humidity. I really began to wonder what the factors were, especially on the organic farms that cannot use regular fly spray. I really think that the three factors mentioned are the key to whether or not pinkeye occurs. Of the three, I think that correct nutrition (as seen by **good body condition**) is the most critical for an animal to be able to fend off infections of all kinds. Parasitism robs nutrition from animals (especially weanlings), so they require more energy in the feed in order to maintain some sort of balance if no conventional wormer is being used.

Prevention

If you are going to vaccinate against pinkeye—and I would strongly recommend considering it for those young animals on pasture that are not handled much—do it prior to mid-June. Remember that vaccines shouldn't be the only avenue of prevention under consideration, but pinkeye vaccinating is one of those management tools that I think all dairy farmers should consider, especially in young stock on pasture that are generally not handled or easily treatable. Sometimes a herd will have problems on a yearly basis. Those herds almost always start vaccinating and now repeat with a yearly booster.

Most vaccines, like MaxiGuard or Piliguard, require only one shot under the skin about four to six weeks prior to pinkeye season. The one I like best is Maxi-Guard by Addison Labs. Although meant for prevention, it has also worked therapeutically as a control measure in animals with very early clinical signs of pinkeye, if given no later than the early "sleepy and weepy" stage. If the infection has continued to the gray haze or further, the vaccine won't stop the infection, especially when the afflicted animals are weanlings in poor body condition, parasitized internally and on crummy pasture, or is a fresh heifer with the stresses of freshening all around.

Fortunately the vaccine is quickly effective after it's given. While vaccinating won't help animals that are currently in the middle of battling pinkeye, it could still help the rest of the animals in those herds where pinkeye is currently hitting—if you vaccinate *without any further delay*. I don't know how to put it more simply than that. The pinkeye vaccine is available from any farm store that has refrigeration, and it's available from three different manufacturers. All brands that I know of instruct to use one shot under the skin. It really can't be made any simpler, yet people will probably still ask if I really think that vaccinating for pinkeye is a good thing to do. Here is the straight-up answer: *yes*.

For pinkeye prevention, of course fly control is critical. This topic is itself a multifactor effort, but for the weanlings out back, a hanging barrel with its own solar panel to trigger a spray of mist onto the animals face as it goes for salt, minerals or other goodies is especially useful for those face flies. The apparatus is called The Protector. As far as sprays go, either regular fly spray, Agri-Dynamics Ecto-Phyte essential oil mix, or PyGanic (pyrethrum) work fairly well but need repeated spraying, often on a near daily basis. I have seen a herd spraying iodine along the bottom midline of cows and their backs and saw extremely few flies on the animals even though it was hot and humid weather. Some people have recommended adding iodine in the water tubs. Kelp (with its iodine) by itself may help to keep the animals in balance but does not seem to help

> **FORTUNATELY THE VACCINE IS QUICKLY EFFECTIVE** after it's given. While vaccinating won't help animals that are currently in the middle of battling pinkeye, it could still help the rest of the animals in those herds where pinkeye is currently hitting– if you vaccinate without any further delay.

clear an active infection once it is started. I'm not certain if kelp is the main item to prevent pinkeye, but it sure should be part of any dairy farm animal ration. That's a no-brainer. As a herdsman in the 1980s we were already using Thorvin kelp at that time. The usual rate for feeding kelp to cows is a minimum of two ounces per head daily up to six ounces per head daily.

Flies are attracted to moisture and will go to animals that look sweaty and glistening. Therefore try to reduce moisture in the animal's environment or upon the animals themselves. Use field lime or diatomaceous earth poured upon the animals' backs via holes punched in an old cow aspirin container. Use *liberally* as needed. This will make animals look dry. One herd where I saw this being done has essentially all white cows, even though they were the standard black and white Holsteins. Another thing to remember is that unclipped pastures can cause grazing cows' eyes to water and attract flies, so clipping pastures would be helpful to prevent pinkeye and to reduce rank growth and give uniform regrowth.

Signs

The very first sign of pinkeye is a "weepy, sleepy" eye with some running, clear drainage. After this phase, if the infection progresses, a gray haze will be seen in one location or throughout the eye.

The next sign will be an eye pinched tightly shut due to the intense pain the animal is feeling. Effective treatment at this point is needed without delay if one is to be kind to their animals. If allowed to continue without treatment, the eye begins a rapid decline towards an angry-looking reddish ring around a thick, solid-white center; then a tiny ulcer may develop on the center of the eye. The eye will slowly recover over a few weeks, or, rarely, it either bursts forth its contents or becomes very enlarged, either which causes permanent blindness in that eye. Normally upon recovery, a slight white "dash" (scar) is seen in the eye and the animal will be able to see around that. The usual time frame for this sequence of events is about five to seven days until the angry "monster eye" appears and another three weeks for it to resolve.

About 90–95 percent of pink eye cases will return to normal and only leave a small white "dash" in the eye.

Treatment

Treating pinkeye can be easy, if you are conventional and can use antibiotics freely. It generally cures with a single intramuscular shot of Bio-Mycin or LA-200 brands of oxytetracycline (4.5cc per hundred pounds, with no more than 12cc at any one spot). If the infection is at a crisis ("monster eye"), having the vet inject the eye with a combination antibiotic, steroid, and atropine can save the eye from rupturing. Even if you do use an antibiotic, animals infected with pinkeye need to be kept out of direct sunlight as sunlight will aggravate the condition. You can certainly let the animals out at night. Alternatively, call the folks at Nasco and get eye patches. These can work pretty well, especially if early.

Treatment of pinkeye if not using antibiotics consists of repeatedly cleansing the eye many times a day with an eyewash for a week or two to keep the infection in check. At this point natural treatments such as sprays of eyebright (*Euphrasia officinalis*) and homeopathic hypericum and aconitum can give good benefit. The best is probably a combination of aqueous calendula tincture spray or 0.9 percent saline spray with multi-potency homeopathic euphrasia, hypericum, and aconite. This is easier for milk cows that can be kept in tie-stalls, compared to free-running yearlings, yet this is *very* labor intensive, obviously. Keep animals inside during the day and let them out for nighttime grazing to avoid ultraviolet rays, which make the condition worse. The eye needs to be sprayed about four times a day.

Once the animal's eye is pinched shut in pain, more drastic treatment is needed. In local organic herds, I have used two different methods. The first is to inject a small amount of hyper-immune plasma or serum (Bovi-Sera or multi-serum) under the first layer of the eye (the cornea), much the same way the conventional combination of penicillin, dexamethasone, and atropine is used. I have seen this stop the infection with a slow but constant, gradual clearing. The corneal injection seems to work best in young stock. The other method is a veterinary procedure, sewing the nictitans (third eyelid) across the entire eyeball and then sewing the eyelids closed together. Absorbable suture is used, which breaks down about twelve to fourteen days later. This method is excellent for any age animal and is a "once-and-done" deal, and the animal can go back outside right away. Since both the delicate intra-corneal injection and the stitching near the eyeball require the animal to remain completely still, excellent restraint with a halter tied tight to a pipe as well as sedation (xylazine) and anesthesia (lidocaine sprayed onto the eyeball) are needed. If using xylazine and lidocaine on an organic cow, an eight-day milk withholding from the tank is required—but the animal will remain organic. The milk held out of the tank can be fed to pre-weaned calves as the source cow is still organic (just not putting her milk in the tank temporarily).

As a reminder, animals with pinkeye are not eligible at the time of pinkeye for state health charts for purposes of sale since pink eye is a contagious infection.

It should seem obvious that preventing pinkeye rather than treating it is the goal. Vaccinating is simply the best way to individually protect animals while reducing fly pressures will also help to make your animals feel more comfortable generally.

CHAPTER 9

Handling the Heat

Is it hot enough for you? Summer can hit hard and fast, and more likely than not there'll be more heat in store as it progresses. I've found over the years that the weather around July 4 somewhat predicts what it will be like the rest of the summer.

Above 80ºF (25ºC) and as humidity increases, we all get to feeling more uncomfortable. How do you keep your animals comfortable in high humidity and high temperature? Remember that while pasture and grazing is great to keep cows healthy, the hottest days of summer are *not* times for dairy cows to be on pasture—they won't graze if they're too hot anyway. Temperatures above 90ºF with low humidity are when cows become uncomfortable, but temperatures as low as 75ºF–80ºF degrees with high humidity will already have cows drop feed intake by a third, causing an associated drop in milk. If cows are waiting at the gate and looking to the barn, they want to come in. Do something; don't just keep them standing there.

While grazing well-managed pastures with their fresh and moisture-containing vegetation may have a cooling effect on the digestive tract of herbivores, direct exposure to an unrelenting sun can offset any benefits of grazing pasture. The same goes for animals housed with poor ventilation if it's hot. Simply put, if animals are too hot and not cooled off in some fashion, they will drop in feed intake and milk production. Heat stress and flat-out heat stroke are always a risk with sunny days above 80°F. Fortunately, over the years, it seems that most farmers have taken appropriate measures to keep cows comfortable during hot weather.

High producers and just-fresh and near-fresh animals will be the first animals in the herd to suffer from heat stress. When the weather is hot, hazy, and humid, cows' nutrient requirements can increase some 15–20 percent simply due to panting, sweating, and urinating. Sweating depletes potassium and urinating depletes sodium, in addition to fluid loss in general. Using the Native Lick can replenish needed minerals.

Your cows may not be as interested in eating when they are panting, but they probably *will* be interested in drinking clean and fresh water. Free access to clean, fresh water is a no-brainer. Do *not* make your cows walk far or search for water! Besides being the most important nutrient in their diet, water is essential to prevent dehydration and keep them cool. The moisture in grazed paddocks is not enough for their needs. Cows will seek water from other sources if you do not provide easy access water in the pasture. When they drink from creeks and puddles, the water quality can be highly questionable. Not only could germs be present (especially in slow-moving water or ponds), but there may also be unwanted chemicals and nitrates. This will definitely stress your cow's internal equilibrium, and if challenged with infection, she may not be able to fight it off. Remember that cows will drink anywhere from ten to thirty gallons of water a day depending on size of animal, stage of lactation and season. A fresh cow in July may easily consume thirty gallons a day, so provide what she needs to keep her cool and producing.

Cows that are too hot may also break with respiratory problems, especially if they had pneumonia as a calf or when transitioning into the fresh string. It always strikes people odd that cows can get pneumonia in the summer time; it's probably due to the opportunistic bacteria that are normal inhabitants of the respiratory tract taking advantage of a stressed cow.

Heat Stroke

Signs of heat stroke are very consistent among animals, it's just that some are more at risk than others: those that are clinically ill, those teetering on becoming ill, and especially those right around calving time.

What is *heat stroke*? The condition involves the increase of body temperature to an extreme point. Unreasonably high temperatures in an animal that seemed completely healthy a few hours ago would be *above* 106°F–107°F. Therefore, on a very hot and humid summer day, it would be wise—indeed, necessary—to check an animal that is down or otherwise depressed to see what her temperature is. Most times, a typical heat stroke will be 106°F–108°F. If the temperature is above 108°F, like 109°F–110°F, the cow (or horse) will either not recover fully or recover at all since that level of temperature causes

Relative Changes in Expected Dry Matter (DMI) and Milk Yield and Water Intake with Increasing Environmental Temperature

Temperature (°F)	DMI (lbs.)	Milk yield (lbs.)	Water intake (gallons)
68	40.1	59.5	18.0
77	39.0	55.1	19.5
86	37.3	50.7	20.9
95	36.8	39.7	31.7
104	22.5	26.5	28.0

Notice this is information is from the National Research Council in 1981. Information like this doesn't change. With increasing heat, cows eat less, milk less, and need more water; it's that simple. Cows need—and will drink—thirty gallons of water a day!*

Sources: National Research Council. 1981. Effect of Environment on Nutrient Requirements of Domestic Animals. National Academy Press, Washington, D.C. Dr. Joe West, Extension Dairy Specialist, University of Georgia.

* An online article by a team of authors from the University of Arkansas provides good information. Jodie A. Pennington and Karl VanDevender, "Heat Stress in Dairy Cattle," University of Arkansas Division of Agriculture Extension, January 2011, http://www.extension.org/pages/11047/heat-stress-in-dairy-cattle#Signs_of_Heat_Stress.

brain damage. Check the temperature of the worst-affected animal to know where she is on the temperature spectrum. On the worst days, normal cows will have elevated temperatures in the range of 103°F or so when they are coming in from pasture or when in the barnyard congregated together. Simple heat stress can deteriorate into heat stroke in animals that have had pneumonia at some point in the past (look in the health record) or in just-fresh older cows with low blood calcium levels.

Difference between Heat Stress and Heat Stroke

A *heat-stressed* cow (or horse) will show signs of open-mouth panting with quick, shallow breathing but can still stand, while a heat-stroke cow will usually be down and not rise. A *heat-stroke* cow will have shallow, rapid respirations and usually appears depressed or even co-matose—much like a milk fever cow. The pupils of the eyes will be dilated. The animal will feel hot to the touch. She may or may not be sweating. If you do a rectal on her, she will feel like she is burning up internally (which she basically is). Heat-stroke animals tend to not drink water, while a heat-stressed animal will. Basically the difference between a heat-stressed cow and a heat-stroke cow is that the heat-stroke cow will have lost control of normal functions (cannot stand, won't drink, nonresponsive, or comatose). Unfortunately, milk-fever cows and coliform-mastitis cows show these signs as well, so you must check the quarters for watery secretions and take into account if she is just fresh and an older cow (suspicious for milk fever/low calcium). The older fresh cows sometimes get "caught" in the sun and can't get out of the area since they are too weak to get up from the milk fever. Treat the milk fever first. It is entirely possible that a cow that started with milk fever or coliform mastitis also develops heat stroke.

Treatment

While milk fever and coliform mastitis are treated in the vein with electrolytes and medicines, heat-stroke and heat-stress animals are primarily treated by hosing down the animal with cold water con-tinuously for twenty to thirty minutes, head to tail, with special attention paid to hosing the back of the head since this is where the cow's temperature regulation center is. (If treating heat stress in pigs, do *not* hose the back of the head.) Heat-stressed cows will often stand still to be hosed down with no need of tying them to anything. Intravenous fluids (five or more liters of lactated ringers solution, 500cc dextrose, and 200cc 8.4 percent sodium bicarbonate) are definitely indicated for heat stroke but are secondary to using a hose. If a hose is not available, quickly move the cow on a four-by-eight-foot plywood board or a tractor bucket to an area where a hose is. Although your intentions may be good, a sponge bath or lugging out a few buckets of cold water and dumping them over the cow will be ineffective. If a cow is deemed to have both milk fever and heat stroke, treat IV for the milk fever (do *not* put oral liquids into the mouth of an animal that is weak and down). When an overly hot animal is hosed down for a good twenty to thirty minutes, the temperature will often drop to about 103°F (just above normal), which is an excellent sign that your hydrotherapy treatment worked.

A **HEAT-STRESSED COW** (or horse) will show signs of open-mouth panting with quick, shallow breathing but can still stand, while a heat-stroke cow will usually be down and not rise. A **HEAT-STROKE COW** will have shallow, rapid respirations and usually appears depressed or even comatose—much like a milk fever cow.

Prevention

While there's not much you can do about the weather, there are things you can do to prevent animals from getting heat stroke. More and more people are misting their cows to cool them, either in the cow yard or at the feed rack. And while I don't think allowing cows in streams is generally a good idea, on the most oppressive hottest days it seems reasonable to let them enjoy some wading time in the water. Allowing cows into the woods is another option. But making them wait at the gate until milking time to come in from a baking pasture is simply being foolish.

We all know how cows can look on a very hot and humid afternoon when they come in to be milked. They can appear rather withered in a sense. Of course they tank up on water. If you see this, you might ask yourself why they are drinking so much all at once. Possibly not enough water is being delivered to them while outside at other times of the day, and/or the water quality available to them is not desirable. It is under these circumstances that animals may be drinking highly objectionable water from little puddles outside in the pastures or from small creeks that slowly wind their way through the landscape and may carry potentially harmful bacteria and parasites. Make sure your cows always have access to fresh, protected water sources.

Some other things to keep in mind are shade and ventilation. For some reason, cows like to bunch together when hot. But if there is enough shade, they will at least disperse into small groups. There is nothing worse for a group of cows than one lone tree they all try to stand under.. A mucky area under one or a couple trees will create more

Watering Tips

When summer has arrived with lots of hot and humid days, let's remember our cows while we are out in the fields. Thinking about water for our animals is always smart.

Here are some tips regarding water quality and animal health:

1. **Provide clean, fresh water—*the* most important nutrient!**
   - Cows can drink up to thirty *gallons* of water each day (depending on production, size, season)
   - If not provided, cows *will* search for water in ditches, puddles, and streams.
   - Monitor quality: nitrates, coliforms. If needed, use peroxide, sand filters, UV light, etc.
   - Monitor quantity: get a water meter if needed
   - Your cows are your income; they deserve lots of good, clean water to keep making lots of milk.
   - Cows *never* get used to bad water.

2. Standing Water Can Harbor Diseases
- Puddles in barnyards contain manure and urine.
  - Salmonella, coliforms, and lepto thrive in puddles and saturated manure.
  - Clinical signs include diarrhea, fever, mastitis, and abortions.
- Saturated manure and moist bedding in pens or stalls are hotbeds for disease.
- Stressed animals (just fresh or high-producing cows) are at increased risk.

3. Slow-Moving Water Carries Diseases with It
- Cows standing in streams are exposed to the problems happening upstream.
- Cows urinating and dropping manure into streams create problems for your neighbors downstream, and we are all, in a sense, "downstream."

4. Warm, Wet Conditions Can Hurt Hooves/Start Mastitis
- Muck and puddles will soften hooves to such an extent that bacteria can enter and gravel can easily puncture the soles, causing abscesses, footrot, and/or strawberry/hairy heel.
- Leaky, heavy producers will have environmental germs (coliforms, strep, and staph) enter the teat canal. This is usually caused by moist bedding in the stall or lying as a group under a tree. The result will be high somatic cell count or actual mastitis.

health problems than no shade at all. On the worst days, in barns with good tunnel ventilation (whether free stall, bedded pack or tie-stall), it is more beneficial to keep the cows in during the day and let them out to graze or exercise at night. It's no sin to keep cows indoors during oppressively hot days. Cows will graze *much* better in the early morning and cooler evenings than during bright daylight hours when it's steaming. Reduce feeding of high carbohydrate/starchy rations (i.e., grains) during hot spells since they tend to "heat up" the rumen generally and replace grains with haylage/grass silage, hay, and evening grazing. Oats are a cooler grain to feed if interested in trying that.

Without doubt, tunnel ventilation provides a much more comfortable environment for both the cows and the workers. Keeping cows in all day without either tunnel ventilation or something nearly like it can make for very uncomfortable cows. Also, having really big cows (heavy body weight and over-conditioned) can make for problems in the summer because of the heat generated internally from metabolism produced from very rich rations. These cows really need tunnel ventilation and/or big fans.

Most intensively grazed cows are not burdened by excess body condition (usually they are too lean if anything), but if they are to get most of their nutrition from pastures, then attention must be paid to their comfort out in the pastures. Cross-bred cows and leaner cows tend to be resilient in the heat compared to big fat ones. It does not matter what the breed is, if an animal is fat, she will suffer in the heat. Many graziers will easily point a finger at Holsteins as being inferior grazing animals, but I take exception to that. One herd I know has about ten out of forty animals of ages twelve and up—the oldest being eighteen and still in the milking herd. The herd is all Holstein. The trick to getting longevity in cows is in their conformation and especially their legs. If you want cows that will last a long time, breed for legs rather than production. And keep them exercised.

Tunnel ventilation, if you have it, also keeps flies from being a problem as they cannot fight the air current. Even if you don't have tunnel ventilation, it may be better for your animals to be taken off pasture during those blazing midday hours, keeping them around the barnyard out of direct sunlight if possible. Most people have a large box fan or overhead fans to help animals keep cool. Since I've driven between farms a lot, I tend to keep my windows down and not use air conditioning, so I get acclimated to the heat in general. Almost universally, getting out of the truck and going into a barn with fans running (whatever sort) always beats no fans or no shade or no breeze. Curtain barns are excellent at catching whatever breeze may be available. Keeping the animals in for the least amount of time is the goal of most graziers. However, keeping animals cooler by keeping them in during the day with whatever fans and practicing nighttime grazing is smartest during the hottest stretches. Portable shades in pasture are helpful as long as there are enough square feet of shade provided for the amount of animals.

A handy hint for calves in hutches is to raise the back of the hutch off the ground during hot days by placing a cinder block there to prop up the back. This will give nice ground flow of air circulation, which will greatly help keeping the animal cool. Simply prop up the back for the rest of the season until it starts cooling down.

Farms that like to graze animals on pasture also need to keep in mind what folks driving by may see in relation to a down cow. The large animal protection officer in my area has gotten in touch with me to treat ailing animals that have been seen by people driving by. As long as the animal receives prompt veterinary attention, the officer will not levy a fine. Preventing any down cows in a field on very hot days is reason enough to bring in the cows in late morning when they are finished grazing so they can be cooled by fans or lots of shade.

Environmental management is a very important skill for farmers to hone. Although we cannot control the weather, we certainly can control the areas our cows inhabit to help prevent potential disasters in the heat of summer.

CHAPTER 10

Weanlings on Pasture

It is common knowledge that cows grazing well-managed pastures will have dramatically fewer general health problems, and especially less digestion problems since they are eating what they were created to eat. The key to fewer health problems, of course, is *well-managed* pastures. Yet young stock, those around the time of weaning and then placed out on pasture, are a slightly different story. As everyone is well aware, young stock six months of age and older must also be eating at least 30 percent dry matter on average from pasture during the entire grazing season. We thus need to balance the environment and nutrition of these more delicate animals before being placed on pasture so they do not succumb to common problems that adult animals tend to fend off better.

A lot depends on how strong the calves are as they are weaned and shortly thereafter. Weaning time is extremely stressful for the calves, regardless of how they were given milk: from an individual bottle in a hutch or if they have been running freely with nurse cows. Weaning may be more stressful to calves having been on nurse cows, but those calves tend to be more robust as well. There are good points and bad points to everything.

Unlike drying off a cow abruptly to get the best results by stopping the brain's signal to make milk, weaning should be done as gradually as possible to avoid stressing calves, especially upsetting their digestion. Prior to weaning, your calves should already be eating *all* the kinds of feed that they soon will be completely reliant on. They should already be used to the forage and grain. Their rumens are functional prior to weaning time, and having forage as part of the feeding routine enhances health of the rumen by keeping a fiber mat for the calves to chew cud, which provides saliva and sodium bicarbonate to help keep the rumen pH at about 6.8, where it should be for the best internal environment for the microbes that live in there. A healthy mat of fiber in the rumen also helps to slow down the rate of passage of feed in general.

Calves fed only grain and milk as pre-weaned animals (a feeding method conjured up by academic research in the 1990s and most likely funded by grain company money) tend to have more digestive upsets and may even experience rumen acidosis, which can affect their ankles and hooves for the rest of their lives (see this by strong pink areas at the ankle). This is a terrible condition at any age but even worse in an animal so young.

Another stress to calves is dehorning/disbudding. Hopefully everyone is now using the portable burners on a regular, periodic basis for different sets of growing calves and not using choppers as a caveman would use on older calves. Using a burner is much, much less stressful than the choppers and also leaves no blood at all, which reduces the attraction for flies and their wiggling, burrowing maggot offspring that can inhabit the chopped site. Make sure when burning that there is a copper-colored ring at the base of the horn bud, usually after seen about five to ten seconds when the burner is good and hot. Do not flick off the now dead horn cap, it will fall off over a couple weeks time. If you do force it off, it could cause bleeding. Still, disbudding even with a burner is stressful and should be done well before weaning, ideally at about one to two months old, and with lidocaine for anesthesia. This of course means you are not weaning until three months old. Do not dehorn (by any method) at the time of weaning or shortly thereafter. Always give a good solid week before weaning. I've seen too many instances when calves are weaned and dehorned during crummy damp weather and the stressed animals come down with pneumonia.

It's not rocket-science to realize that a cow's milk is meant for her offspring calf. The biological signal for peak milk production of dairy cows starts to decrease at two to three months into lactation. Once the calves reach three months of age or older they need less milk and rely mainly on solid food. Calves will naturally be stronger the longer they are on milk, which will translate into animals that can weather the common problems that occur when they are weaned and put on pasture. But with the current grazing requirements for animals six months of age and older, you now have to tend to this group of animals in regards to pasture management almost as closely as your milking cows.

By rearing a healthy, robust calf, underlying problems such as low levels of parasites encountered on pasture will not be quite as much of an issue. You need to be aware that as you put calves out on pasture in the summer, there are stomach worm larvae waiting there to meet them from the last season if young stock were out there the last grazing season. As the warmth and humidity of spring and summer go on, the stomach worm larvae population will increase dramatically, so you really need to make sure that calves are receiving proper levels of energy, protein and minerals for their immune systems to mature quickly enough while the animals are encountering these pests for the first time. A young local farmer had a fantastic idea of putting the young animals on the pasture for a few days and then take them away for about a month, and then put them

> **IT'S NOT ROCKET-SCIENCE TO REALIZE THAT A COW'S MILK IS MEANT FOR HER OFFSPRING CALF.** The biological signal for peak milk production of dairy cows starts to decrease at two to three months into lactation.

on it for real. Without realizing it, the young farmer was applying a concept of vaccination in a very natural way: expose an animal to a low amount of challenge, withdraw for three weeks for the immune system to process the incoming information, and then reexpose the animal to trigger the immune system to the fullest.

If calves born in February through April and weaned three months later are sent out back to the same paddock where such groups of animals always go, they will quickly become infested with internal stomach worms since they have no natural immunity to them. Typical signs of infestation include pot-bellied calves with obvious angularity to observable bones, a rough-looking and reddish-black coat, with diarrhea and dried manure on thin back legs. Animals in the age group between one month after weaning up to about ten to twelve months old are the most likely to become infested. Once past this age, they tend to have enough wherewithal to build a solid, natural immunity that will be with them for life. See chapter 10 for more information on parasites.

If any part of their nutritional needs is not met, however, even the best calves will start to look worse and worse over the course of the pasture season. I have seen this occur way too often over the years. But to be fair I have also seen really nice calves their first season on pasture, *if* they are fed properly and the pasture is managed such that it is not a wasteland of rank forage growth with more weeds than actual forage.

Clipping Pastures

Okay, so besides proper feeding, what are some basic management procedures to keep in mind for young animals during their first year on pasture? The thing that immediately comes to mind is *clipping pastures*. I have seen many pastures filled with orchard grass gone to head and becoming brownish. First, this means that the plants have lignin and are less usable. Second, these rank, brown stands will potentially prick and irritate calves' eyes as they seek out the softer, greener vegetation lower down. Third, valuable real estate is being wasted. Fourth, and especially with orchard grass, once the plants have headed out, any regrowth (even after clipping) is less palatable due to chemical changes that have taken place within the plant as it went to seed. Thus the potential utilization of that paddock when grazed again will be diminished significantly.

Clipping pastures is a primary method of ensuring uniform regrowth as well as cutting down weeds that might be heading out soon.

Pre-Clipping

On one farm where I was walking the pastures with the farmer, the pastures were a thick, green carpet with no stalky weeds. The cows looked great as far as body condition. I asked the farmer what he was doing. He said he was clipping the pasture *before* the cows graze it. He started this practice in early August when it was blasted hot—and the cows went up in milk! The cows eat everything in sight since it is all clipped and softer due to wilting. They loved it and cleaned it right up. Such a simple management tool has powerful effects. Think of it, all that fescue, burdock, quackgrass, redroot pigweed, and foxtail all mixed in with the clover, orchard grass, and alfalfa. A true pasture total mixed ration! The clipping should be done about two to six hours prior to grazing the paddock. Use a standard disc mower or sickle bar—don't use a mower conditioner. It is probably best suited for the time of the year when common pasture species slow down and the "weeds" come up. Remember that those "weeds" do have nutritional value. Many exceed the nutritional standard of alfalfa. Moreover, they have medicinal value that animals can sense, it seems, as you see them eat quite a variety of plants when walking them in from pasture or looking at what they've nibbled on in a pasture they were just in. Maybe they just want a variety of tastes and textures. Who knows, but providing a variety of plants for an herbivore to eat is always good. And with clipping beforehand, they do eat everything. It was really amazing and I am still blown away by how simple yet powerful a management tool it is. If you've been against clipping pasture for one reason or another, give it some thought. It could well change the way you graze forever. You will be maximizing your animals' pasture intake, thereby naturally feeding them much more effectively. Hey, this may even reduce your need for grain since they will be taking in more dry matter and energy.

While I have always been a big fan of clipping pastures if only to have uniform regrowth, timing the clipping for after animals have been in a pasture is important. Ideally, a pasture should be clipped at day three after grazing. Why? Two reasons: dung beetles and horn flies. Dung beetles break down the organic matter of manure quickly so that stomach worm larvae do not build up. They do most of their work within the first two days after the fresh manure has been deposited. Earthworms help to incorporate that organic matter into the soil as well. Also within the first two days of fresh manure being deposited, horn flies will land and lay eggs for the next generation of flies to come into being. Waiting two days prior to clipping will allow the dung beetles to do their job and give the horn flies time to lay their eggs, which will then be eradicated by the mowing. Alternatively to mowing, you can drag the manure with chains behind your tractor so it spreads out and dries up more quickly with sun and wind. Drying it out will harm the stomach worm larvae that quickly hatch out of their relatively strong shells. A biological way to reduce manure patties is with chickens. Their natural action of scratching and pecking destroys manure patties quite well. Whichever way you choose to help manure patties disintegrate, always wait two days, until the beneficial dung beetles have done their job and the horn flies have laid their eggs.

Timely clipping to a residual height of three to four inches will steadily increase the value of your pastures. Ideally, animals should be placed into the pastures when the height of clover is seven to eight inches and some bloom, any alfalfa is ten to twelve inches and early bloom, and grasses are twelve to eighteen inches tall and early head. These heights are for any age animal as the Brix (sugar/energy) is highest at this

> **WHILE I HAVE ALWAYS BEEN A BIG FAN OF CLIPPING PASTURES** if only to have uniform regrowth, timing the clipping for after animals have been in a pasture is important. Ideally, a pasture should be clipped at day three after grazing.

stage also. If much higher, consider pre-clipping paddocks a couple hours prior to placing animals in them. This will wilt the clippings, and the animals tend to devour everything rather than leaving areas untouched. Proper pasture management is not only legally required now for organics, it is smart use of resources within the perimeter of your farm as well as a healthy way not only to feed cows but young stock as well.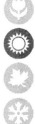

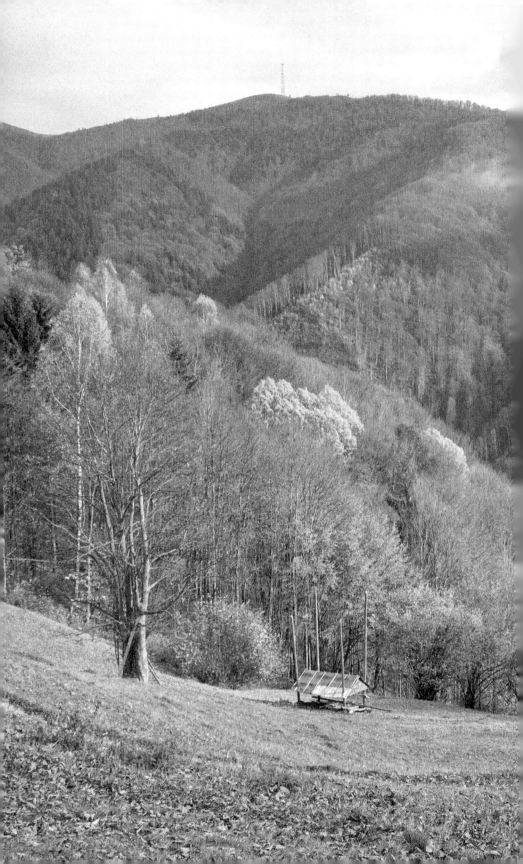

PART III
Fall

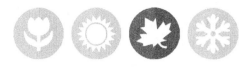

CHAPTER 11

Vaccinations

As the summer season draws to a close, consider how your animals have done out on pasture. As I've written, adult cows generally can withstand various environmental pressures that younger animals simply cannot. Younger animals don't have the ability to adjust as well to brand new situations since their immune systems have not had previous exposure to various challenges yet. This is where vaccinating for a disease that has repeatedly occurred on a farm may be beneficial. While vaccines will prepare an animal for future challenges, some farmers can rely on them too much and can conceal some root cause of disease in the animals' environment. Additionally, vaccines won't work well if the animals' nutritional plane is deficient.

One thing to think about is animal concentration—what is the optimal number of animals to have for a certain size of land or barn? That's a real question. The beautiful stone barns of the southeastern Pennsylvania countryside were originally meant to house no more than probably fifteen cows, their young stock, a few horses, and a handful of pigs and chickens. Now they routinely house forty or more cows, some young stock, and a full team of horses. I think it only makes sense that when there is a high density of animals in one area, bugs and germs have an easier time setting up shop in the animals there. That's why routine massive vaccination programs have become so common place in modern agriculture—because of the high concentration of animals in one location, whether it is a forty- to fifty-cow tie stall in a stone barn or a four hundred– to four thousand–cow free-stall system.

I am not strongly in favor of vaccination, nor am I opposed to vaccination—it all depends on factors within an individual farm. While vaccinating prevents disease, I think that it's also a crutch that allows for an unnaturally high density of animals to be kept together. Vaccines certainly can prevent terrible diseases—thank God for the rabies vaccine. There have been no alternative forms of prevention for rabies. Unvaccinated people or animals bitten by a rabid animal will die unless they get the antibody treatment in time. (See Chapter 20 on rabies.) On the other hand, some vaccines seem to be weak, evidenced by the need for one to two shots a year. One would think that a truly good vaccine would provide long-standing immunity, hopefully for many years. For example, the rabies vaccine in people is good for five to ten years, and in most small animals it's good for three years. I'm definitely not in favor of excessive vaccination programs as it may confuse the immune system or possibly create a tolerance effect, which is when the body becomes accustomed to the injected material and no longer mounts a response.

As the saying goes, an ounce of prevention is worth a pound of cure. It all comes down to priorities, ideals, and reality—not always an easy set of factors to balance in farming situations with multi-factorial causes to problems. But keep trying, it'll be worth it in the long run.

To Vaccinate or Not?

Do we need to vaccinate if we are abiding by the "high-forage diet, fresh air, and dry bedding" rule? That depends on some factors.

Respiratory Bugs

The first thing to consider is what you want to vaccinate against. Is it the respiratory bugs mainly? It's a common practice to do so. In some ways doing so admits that indoor living isn't as good as the outdoors on pasture, right? I have come to realize that, truly, the best vaccination program is one that is based on fresh air, high-forage diets, and dry bedding—at least for respiratory health. Another important way to prevent respiratory problems in stabled animals is to put them outside every day for as long as possible. This allows them to breathe in fresh air every day. Remember that most dairy cattle breeds are from northern European climates and like temperatures between 20°F–50°F (-5°C–10°C). There is no need to keep them inside when it is 22°F if the sun is shining, there is little wind, and the footing is not slippery. The absolute worst possible weather for cattle to be outside is when it's raining and barely above freezing. They will lose body condition fast. If young stock are carrying an internal parasite burden, or if they have poor body condition due to insufficient feed and energy intake, they will likely break with pneumonia in such weather conditions. Young stock with such issues may also break with pneumonia when put inside, especially if the bedding becomes damp, there is a draft at ground level, and they are in a cinder block or wooden building with no fresh air.

If this housing situation is unavoidable, then vaccinating with one of the intranasal vaccines (InForce 3) that protects against the typical respiratory viruses like BRSV, PI3, and IBR is best as it gives quick protection within a few days and will last a few months. I have always liked the idea of the intranasal vaccines if only because they mimic the real way respiratory germs typically gain entrance to the body—through the nose. Otherwise, buildings with excellent air movement just above the height of the animals but allowing no drafts at bedding level (such as curtain barns, hoop houses, or large super hutches) are great for keeping weaned animals and bred heifers in.

Reproductive Bugs

If vaccinating is for reproductive bugs, then you may want to consider what kind of specific reproductive problems, if any, have been occurring. There will always be a few cows that don't settle easily. What about cows called pregnant around days thirty-five through forty of pregnancy that then come back into heat a month later? Or actual abortions seen—how many, in what size herd, and during what time span? In a fifty-cow herd, it's not unreasonable to see one spontaneous abortion over a year, or maybe two if they are far apart. If you see two to three abortions in a fifty-cow herd within a month or two, I would start wondering what is going on. Typically, cows that abort at one to three months pregnant may be challenged by bovine viral diarrhea (BVD), at four to six months pregnant they may be challenged by BVD or leptospirosis, and at six to eight months pregnant they may be challenged by neosporosis, caused by *Neospora caninum*. And if many cows are showing irregular heat cycles or perhaps have been bred but come back in heat not on a twenty-one-day cycle, BVD could be an issue.

If a cow aborts, testing the aborted calf and taking two blood samples from the cow (at time of abortion and three weeks later) will give the best possible information for a lab to work with. Or, if there are no abortions but irregular heats or cows not settling, then drawing blood from at least 10 percent of the animals in the herd (testing the problem animals) can reveal what the problem may be. While an aborted fetus is looked at under the microscope and samples are taken to identify any bugs that may be present, blood samples from cows are generally checked for antibodies to challenges. Antibodies to germs like leptospirosis, IBR, BVD, and neospora reveal to what degree the cow's immune system has responded to a challenge from those bugs. The results are presented as titers. Titers numerically show to what degree an animal's immune system has responded to a challenge. Typically, blood is diluted further and further until a response is no longer seen. The higher the titer, the more likely that the bug causing the titer was involved with the problem. However, if you have a vaccinated herd and take blood tests to see what the titers are, those results could affected by the vaccine since vaccines mimic natural exposure and cause the animal's immune system to respond. This is good when the animals are truly exposed to the real bug. Their immune system, if previously primed by a vaccine, is ready to neutralize the challenge immediately. Looking at the titers of animals that haven't been vaccinated in a number of years is very useful because results showing any high titers will indicate that the animals have seen the real challenge by the bugs themselves and are reacting to them.

Be aware that trying to vaccinate your way out of a problem may or may not work. For example, vaccination is a reasonably good idea if Lepto hardjo-bovis bacteria are involved, as that Lepto hardjo-bovis (any kind of lepto) is difficult to get rid of, especially if you're trying not to use antibiotics. But if bovine viral diarrhea (BVD) is floating around in a herd, vaccinating may give a false sense of security. Why? Because a persistently infected (PI) BVD animal may be present. These PI animals are born with BVD after becoming infected with it during gestation if the dam was challenged by BVD in her environment by other cows. Every moment a BVD PI animal is alive they are breathing out, urinating, manuring, and coughing out live BVD particles into the environment that no vaccine can overcome. These animals must be identified and removed from the herd before any BVD vaccine will work to prevent any such future occurrence. See more about BVD in chapter 16.

If vaccinating, using a modified live version (versus a killed version) has proven to be a more effective method of protection. I have read that some immunologists say giving a modified live vaccine against respiratory viruses at six months of age and then again a month before breeding age may give lasting immunity for life. If you think about it, a tetanus vaccine is good for ten years. If vaccinated for measles and mumps, the immunity lasts nearly a lifetime. So why do people vaccinate cattle every year? Well the box says so. Perhaps some studies need to be done to determine how long titers stay high from vaccines, but don't expect vaccine manufacturers to do the studies.

Does an "open herd" (one that has cattle coming into the herd regularly) have potentially more natural immunity to challenges than a "closed herd" (one with no additions and high biosecurity)? Yes—but challenges can be very potent, and therefore vaccinating open herds is usually a smart move. Is any herd ever truly "closed"? If cattle dealers, animal haulers, and nutritionists come onto the farm without using sanitizer on their boots before they leave (if not, then they didn't wash up at the last farm either), or even if you just buy just one bull every other year, your herd is *not* a closed herd.

Are there alternatives to vaccinating? Again, the best "alternative" to vaccinating is likely a solid framework promoting basic healthful living. Autogenous vaccines can also serve as a true alternative to commercial vaccines. Autogenous vaccines are vaccines made right from your own herd and are highly specific to whatever is challenging your herd in particular. I have seen it work very well in a herd continually challenged by *Staphylococcus aureus* mastitis. By vaccinating animals at six months of age and at a year old, first-calf heifers coming fresh with *Staph. aureus* have been reduced from an average of five to six out of ten down to zero to one out of ten freshening. They are then vaccinated yearly about a month prior to the next calving. It took about three years for this beneficial effect to be seen. And that was with no other measures taken.

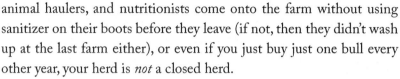

ARE THERE ALTERNATIVES TO VACCINATING?

Again, the best "alternative" to vaccinating is likely a solid framework promoting basic healthful living. Autogenous vaccines can also serve as a true alternative to commercial vaccines.

Homeopathic nosodes are sometimes used as alternatives. To what extent they are truly effective against hot challenges is open to speculation since only one real study, on kennel cough, has ever been done. Remember that anything will appear to work if there is no actual challenge. Maybe your feeding and housing practices are so good that they are the main factor preventing disease, not the homeopathic nosode. But maybe it's both things working together! The real proof is when a hot challenge occurs—a good example is animals being shipped, mingled with yours, and kept together indoors during the winter. One thing for sure is that using homeopathic nosodes will not overload the immune system or create tolerance, as they don't work in the same way vaccines do (animals exposed to nosodes do not produce antibody titers). Nosodes are very safe to give, but truly effective protection is an open question. Real homeopaths will tell you that nosodes are to be used only *during* a disease outbreak, as they are derived from actual disease material. Homeopathy does not generally put forth preventives, other than the pillars of health that I often mention: sound nutrition, clean and dry bedding, fresh air, etc.

I do think vaccines can be abused and harm the immune system if given excessively. I don't quite understand how we humans can get a tetanus shot that lasts for ten years or a rabies vaccine that lasts five to ten years, but almost all the animal vaccines have instructions for revaccinating annually. Can't they improve the vaccines? To be sure, there are many alternative veterinary medicine friends of mine (small animal and equine vets) that take a blood sample to check the protection level (titer) to see whether revaccination is necessary. Maybe that's something farmers should consider before revaccinating as well?

What about not vaccinating at all? If everything has been fine *and* you have all the foundational pillars of health in place *and* you aren't buying in animals *and* whoever visits your farm has sanitized boots, then it should be okay. Always remember this: keeping your animals in robust health by proper feeding, frequent exercise, allowing them to choose to go outdoors or stay inside, and clean and dry bedding is the first step in any immunization program.

Remember that the animals' environment and feed play a much bigger part in staying healthy than vaccines. I'm not against vaccines, but the best "vaccine" for farm animals will always be fresh air, dry bedding, high-forage diets, and sunshine.

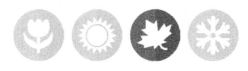

CHAPTER 12

Feed Changes, Digestive Upset and Twisted Stomach

As the effective grazing season draws down with the coming of fall, we need to think about feeds, housing, contented cows, and their immune systems. As I'm not a trained professional nutritionist, I won't be talking about the details of ration formulation, but keep in mind that fresh grazing grass has an enormous amount of living vitality that stored feeds simply do not. This living vitality of fresh-grazed pastures has positive effects on the immune system of animals, if only from the dynamic characteristics of actively growing plants rooted directly to the soil and delivering up minerals that are essential to proper enzyme function within the immune system. Cows out on pasture tend to be healthy—a direct consequence of the fresh feed itself as well as the exercise cows get walking the landscape. Once cows are taken off pasture and fed ensiled feeds and stored hay while staying in the barn, problems can and do happen more frequently. Let's look more closely.

While every farmer feeds their cows differently, those feeding a higher grain diet (which produces proprionic acid in the rumen) tend to see more milk but also more health problems with the cows than those farmers feeding higher forage diets with higher effective fiber intake (which produces acetic acid in the rumen). The safest way to feed cows in the winter is maximal feeding of top-quality dry hay (that has good protein content *as well as* energy—always check the relative feed value and relative feed quality of hay). A good energy feed is one in which the net energy for lactation (NE_L) is 0.65 and higher.

First we should remember that the change to stored feeds and less exercise will impact the immune system. In organics, there is always talk of maintaining a healthy immune system in order to fight off potential germs that the animals may have to deal with. And, even if you can use antibiotics without restriction, an antibiotic is effective only if the animal's immune system is functional. The antibiotic is simply knocking back the bacterial assault, allowing more time for the animal's immune system to rally and overcome the problem. In the end, the animal always needs to rely on her own immune system to maintain and ultimately restore itself to health. I believe, however, that constant, repetitive use of antibiotics and hormones for every problem will slowly weaken the animals over time—even over generations—and give rise to antibiotic resistance. This is where one difference in cow health is evident on conventional versus organic farms: the need to keep an organic animal's immune system at its highest possible level at all times. But even then, there could be an overwhelming germ that for whatever reason slips into the system and causes problems.

Also remember that a cow's rumen needs about two weeks to fully adjust to new feed ingredients. That's right—two weeks. No farmer that I know of ever changes over to a new feed so gradually, but if you want the least disturbance to the routine, that's what you should do. The rumen bugs are adjusted to a certain feed intake, and new feeds change rumen environment and pH, which will kill some rumen bugs but enhance others. Therefore the more gradual the transition of feed stuff, the less the cows in the herd will be negatively be affected. The usual situation is that the farmer finishes up some feed commodity and then simply opens up a new ag-bag or silo and begins feeding it out at the next feeding time in the full amount. To buffer against such a drastic feed change, either feed some extra dry hay or extra probiotics to help the rumen bacteria and protozoa stay as healthy as possible. Or do both.

Fresh cows will have the hardest time with feed changes, since they are adjusting to rapidly increasing milk production as well. Often, the worst offending material is bagged haylage (chopped and not long fiber). Any product (but especially bagged it seems), if not ensiled correctly, will cause watery scours. To help cows adapt more easily, it is good to begin (or step up) feeding a probiotic product with various lactobacillus bugs. Better yet is to make sure that the feed being blown into the bag at harvest time is inoculated with a commercial probiotic to ensure proper pH for fast fermentation. (Make sure the product is allowed if you are certified organic.) If a cow is already scouring, do not feed her *any* type of ensiled feed for twenty-four to forty-eight hours. Feed only grass or mixed grass/alfalfa dry hay along with two cups of uncooked oats twice daily (with molasses). A pill or gel form of a probiotic is good too. Remove her from pasture if scouring (the only time I am against a cow on pasture). The health and immune system of any living being—cow, horse, or human—always starts in the digestive process. If there is digestive upset, there won't be health.

Cows Going Off Feed

A cow "off-feed" is obvious to any observant farmer, but catching it when it just begins can prevent numerous problems from worsening. Some common reasons that a cow goes off-feed include fever, retained placenta, moldy feed, sudden feed changes, diarrhea (scours), and/or ketosis.

Mold

It's no surprise seeing mold in the feed after a particularly wet summer with mold already showing on standing corn plants in the field. Moldy feed usually is associated with ensiled feeds; if you see a chunk of mold in any ensiled feed, chances are very high it is throughout the entire area. I have seen a fair amount of corn smut (*Ustilago maydis*) in my time as well—this is a fleshy growth usually found on the stems and leaf node areas (from what I've seen). Moldy feed can quickly ruin a

> If cows are being pushed for maximal milk production and are recently fresh, there is a possibility that they are on the verge of acidosis if not being fed enough fiber.

herd's milk production due to digestive upset while it is being fed and unfortunately can negatively affect reproduction for even a longer period of time until the molds are fully out of the cows' system. You really need to use a binder that the cows eat right along with the questionable feed, like Dyna-min (from Agri-Dynamics), which binds the molds so they pass harmlessly through the animal's gut without robbing it of its essential nutrients. Of course you should not be feeding any questionable feed to begin with, but sometimes it is unavoidable or simply too late when first observed.

If spoiled feed is an issue, check your cow's temperature if she is scouring (has diarrhea). Place the thermometer *in the vulva* to get an accurate reading. Fever *and* scours, especially if some bloody scours, can indicate an infectious process like salmonella, which can affect others in the herd. Separate the suspect cows and keep them away from other farm animals to minimize the spreading of disease by shared water bowls and feed areas. Any area splattered with manure should be sanitized with Clorox. Once an area is cleaned up, lay down limestone to change the pH, which upsets the bad environmental bugs. Milk from the bulk tank should not be consumed by people if an animal is diagnosed with salmonella as it is contagious to humans.

Ketosis

Ketosis is found in cows that are milking well but all of a sudden go off-feed for whatever reason and subsequently don't take in enough energy through their feed. Cows can also get ketosis as a side effect of a twisted stomach when the stomach is ballooned and they simply don't want to eat. Cows with primary ketosis will have firm manure, look somewhat "sleepy," and typically not be interested in their grain, which is exactly what they actually need for its energy. Ketosis can cause displaced abomasums (DA) by a cow slowing down so much that her digestive motility slows down. Gas is not propelled as it normally should be and builds up, giving rise to a ballooned abomasum (twisted stomach).

Other Feed Change Problems
Acidosis, Hemorrhagic Bowel Syndrome, and Clostridium
If cows are being pushed for maximal milk production and are recently fresh, there is a possibility that they are on the verge of acidosis if not being fed enough fiber. Any further major changes in the diet could send them into a subclinical acidosis with a consequent shift in microorganisms in the lower gut. There are some theories as to the causes of deadly hemorrhagic bowel syndrome (HBS), one being that there is a microorganism (and possibly a specific mold) that is usually present when the animal is checked at post-mortem. Clostridium Type A often seems to be found in animals with HBS. Clostridial organisms are normal inhabitants of the gut and are kept in a delicate balance when there is healthy rumen and abomasum activity. When, however, there is a drop in pH in the gut environment (due to grain fermenting in the gut rather than in the rumen), it is possible that the delicate balance is upset, and this allows the amplification of the Clostridium Type A to overtake the local environment and cause rapid death. Therefore, as I usually mention, it is never wrong to feed extra dry hay as it ensures a good rumen fiber mat so the new feed doesn't go unnecessarily fast through the rumen into the small intestine and cause major negative impact to the intestinal bugs.

Scours
Scours usually are watery, very profuse, and contain undigested feed. The most susceptible cows are those under the most stress—fresh or at peak lactation. If the animal is not dehydrated, determining treatment is simple: put some high-quality dry hay in front of her and see if she will eat. If she digs into it like any normal cow would, that's the treat-

ment. Do *not* feed corn silage or other ensiled feeds to scouring cows; it's like adding fuel to the fire. If you for some reason absolutely cannot feed dry hay, then top-quality, long-fiber grass silage can possibly substitute, as long as the corn silage is kept away. I usually recommend this type of "feed treatment" for a few days until the manure becomes more regular. Then, *slowly* begin to add in the other components. I find that cows normally fed TMR really love extra dry hay thrown to them, even if they are pretty much "on feed." I think this may be due to the particle length as-fed to the cows being too short in many TMR-fed barns. The cows' instinctive need for fiber makes them go for dry hay when offered. The same is true when cows are on lush pasture; they often will even eat straw if offered in order to satisfy their need for a certain minimum of effective fiber intake. Many of my farmers know that one of my main treatments any time a cow is somewhat off-feed or scouring is to feed that particular cow as much hay as she wants for at least a few days. Whole herds probably would have healthier rumens if more hay was fed in general. Healthy rumens make for healthy cows.

If the cow is totally off-feed and has a really watery diarrhea, then we need to support her digestive tract by pumping her stomach with fluids and protectants. The most commonly used protectant is mineral oil. I use one gallon when I pump it in. Like in a horse with colic, it is a lubricant, but, more importantly for a case of diarrhea, it will cap the excess fermentation taking place in the small intestine as well as line the gut so toxins aren't being reabsorbed into the animal's system. Mineral oil is not absorbed by the intestine at all and, though it may sound odd, stays technically external to the animal as it passes through its system.

Another product that works very well, either in addition to mineral oil or given alone, is activated charcoal. Activated charcoal is not the charcoal most farmers think of; it is a processed product made from vegetable sources that helps adsorb (like a magnet) toxins to help pass them out of the animal without them being absorbed. These two items will often stop the cycle of diarrhea quickly without "stopping up" the animal and retaining toxins that are better released. If the animal is dehydrated (you can tell by squeezing the eyebrow and seeing if it stays pinched up after letting go; the longer it stays pinched up, the worse the dehydration) then IV replacement fluids will be needed. A fresh cow milking well will probably need this IV treatment more quickly than a non-stressed animal. I like to give a few liters of lactated ringers solution as well as dextrose, calcium, and hypertonic saline. There is an old saying that giving a gallon of fluids into the vein is worth ten gallons given in the rumen. Probably best is when both are given.

The moral of the story is that when you go through a feed change, no matter how abrupt, feed a bunch of extra dry hay to the cows for about a week, until the rumen bugs have had time to adapt to the new diet. Also, use Dyna-Vites (Agri-Dynamics) to provide probiotics to the rumen.

Twisted Stomach

Feverish cows, especially with a retained placenta and uterine infection early in lactation, are especially prone to getting a twisted stomach (displaced abomasum/DA). These cows look like they feel miserable, depending on the severity of the uterine infection. Cows early in lactation with fever due to bacterial pneumonia usually do not end up getting DAs even though they are off-feed. Cows that are slightly off-feed just prior to calving, especially those older cows that may be deficient in calcium, are likely to get a DA after they calve as there is a lot of empty space in the abdomen for the abomasum to float out of place. Fevers due to hardware may actually lessen the likelihood of a DA since the infection can often lead to scarring of the stomach to the body wall, effectively keeping the abomasum tacked down but forever after hindering general gut motility (periodic bloating usually occurs).

Any problem at the time of calving can make a DA more likely, especially in first-calf heifers that are also entering the feed ration of the milking string for the first time. Typical problems would be calving early and not cleaning (not passing the fetal membranes), twins (almost always leads to some degree of retained placenta), a hard calving (internal pain relief biochemicals block tha natural oxytocin release that would normally help contract the uterus to help push out the placenta), and low calcium levels in older cows or low selenium levels in areas with deficient selenium. These are all "obstetrical" causes of a DA (the cow never gets a good start in lactation from the moment of calving).

The other type of DA is caused primarily by poor feed management. This is when excess grain is being fed relative to fiber and grain escapes the rumen (rather than being trapped in the rumen fiber mat) and goes on to ferment in the abomasum, causing the gas which makes the abomasum float up out of place. In this case, the DA is what I call a "nutritional" DA, one that is not at all due to obstetrics problems but rather to an unbalanced ration.

What exactly is a "displaced" abomasum? The condition simply refers to when the fourth stomach, the abomasum (the true stomach, just like ours), fills with gas and floats from its normal position on the floor of the belly up to the left side and gets pinned between the rumen and the ribcage (LDA) or up to the right (RDA), just beneath the ribs on that side. There is a characteristic "ping" that can be heard when striking your finger upon the ribs while you have your ear on the cow or are using a stethoscope. The ping may sound like a basketball bouncing or a bell chime. Most DAs float up to the left (when looking at the cow from the rear, your left is her left), especially in the first month of lactation—mainly because there is room to do so since the calf no longer takes up belly space and the rumen is not yet filled to capacity. RDAs are more rare, which is fortunate because they can be deadly (due to the anatomy of the right side of the abdomen which can allow the abomasum to twist twice). Please be aware that either kind of DA can happen at any time in the life of a ruminant (cow, bull, calf, goat, sheep, etc.) but that RDAs seem to be more common later in lactation when most farmers aren't thinking about the possibility of a twisted stomach anymore. In my experience, some kind of feed problem (mold) usually causes these late lactation RDAs. Unfortunately, since most farmers don't suspect an RDA, the animal receives supplements and continues to deteriorate until very weak and emergency surgery needs to be done, if it is still possible at all. Learn to listen for pings.

Typical treatment for a DA is surgery. Less common is to roll a cow, and even less commonly cows are culled due to a DA. DAs seem to be part of modern, confinement dairy farming. However, I have wondered sometimes why is it that beef cows don't really get DAs as dairy cows do. All I can figure is that they roam freely over the pasture with their calf when fresh and they are fed mainly forages instead of rapidly increasing amounts of highly fermentable carbohydrate feeds like dairy cows are to make lots of milk. Of course, beef cattle don't produce much. Backing up this hypothesis is my observation that the rate of DAs is extremely low on farms that practice intensive grazing. Normally cows with a retained placenta and associated fever tend to develop DAs, but not so on grazing farms. Cows with even the worst uterus infections (basically festering cesspools) seem to be able to "graze it off" if allowed. Of course, these animals are not highly productive during those first two to three weeks, but they truly seem resilient and able to fend off the predictable DA that otherwise typically develops in cows confined inside and fed a TMR.

> **NORMALLY COWS WITH A RETAINED PLACENTA AND ASSOCIATED FEVER** tend to develop DAs, but not so on grazing farms. Cows with even the worst uterus infections (basically festering cesspools) seem to be able to "graze it off" if allowed.

So, how best to prevent a twist? Get the rumen quickly bulked up with roughages after calving and graze a cow that had calving problems. Do not make rapid feed changes in your cows. I like to use a botanical mix that, if given before a "ping" is heard, has prevented a number of cases that I think would have gone on to become DAs. The mix is fluid extract of ginger, gentian, licorice, peppermint, and tincture of nux vomica. I call it Eat Well. It has been effective in "slow" cows, not eating quite right but not yet twisted. I label it for mildly bloated cows, constipated cows, and also for horse colic. It is based on an old-fashioned horse colic remedy that veterinarians used back in the 1930s. I'm happy to relay that plant medicines such as fluid extracts and tinctures seem to be effective methods in helping our herbivore friends—especially with digestive and liver issues.

As I've always said, you can never feed enough dry hay to dairy cows—it's always okay to feed dry hay. Indeed, feeding even a little dry hay during feeding transitions will help digestion, and thus their immune system. Truly, if we can create a balance between God's design of a cow as a true ruminant and her will to milk, we will maintain healthy and productive animals. You might want to keep this in mind as you transition to winter feeds over the next couple months.

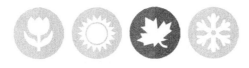

CHAPTER 13

Fall Breeding

Now that we are in the autumn months, fertility usually returns. The mild fall weather helps the cows show heat again. After a really hot spell, the open cows seem to begin cycling again. When I do repro exams at this time of the year, I often find a fair amount of animals within herds that exhibit good uterine "tone"—meaning the uterus is very well defined and has good contractility, which usually means that a cow is near heat or in heat. This is great if you haven't seen the cow in heat for a while but not so good if you thought she was already bred. Breeding cows when it's easier in October and November will have them calve during July and August—right during the usual hot spell stretch. But if cows are long open, they *do* need to get bred back—just try not to have a large percentage of your herd all bred in the late fall.

Knowing that a cow is near heat is obviously important for those of you doing artificial insemination. Traditionally, it was thought that you should wait to perform artificial insemination (AI) for twelve hours after you see the cow in heat. This practice was based partially on the biology of the cow, since it's known that the egg is released from the dominant follicle *after* the cow shows heat. The research that really

IN OTHER WORDS, when you see a cow in heat, you should breed her within twelve hours, preferably six to eight hours. Another way to think about— would a bull wait twelve hours?

propelled the idea of the a.m.–p.m. breeding routine was done in the 1940s, with cows being observed three times daily for signs of heat. Once they observed heat, researchers checked the cow every two hours for further activity, then insemination times were recorded and success rates were evaluated and compared.

The onset of heat (estrus) is very important because the egg will be released at some point afterward. The egg is freshest at the time of release from the follicle and ages over the hours. If watching for heat six times a day, the onset of heat can be detected fairly accurately. But most farmers don't watch this often—they maybe watch twice a day at most. Nowadays, on total confinement herds, breeding programs based solely on injections rather than visual observations are normal. It may take anywhere from three to six injections of hormones to have a cow conceive in the time span that conventional herds require. If, though, cows are observed twice a day for signs of heat, then the farmer really doesn't know when the onset of heat/estrus takes place, and breeding should be done sooner rather than later to take advantage of the freshest timing for the egg. In other words, when you see a cow in heat, you should breed her within twelve hours, preferably six to eight hours. Think about it: if you happen to see the cow during her very last standing heat behavior and then wait twelve hours, you could easily be too late and not get the best timing for the egg being released. Another way to think about—*would a bull wait twelve hours?* So maybe we should observe nature and follow it a bit more closely instead of simply being "traditional." But hey, if your AI breeding is going just fine, don't change anything. But if you feel that you are having too many cows returning to heat, perhaps breeding them sooner would be worth considering.

There certainly can be other reasons for cows returning to heat when they have been bred previously, other than poor AI timing. For instance, in bull-bred herds, if there are many repeats, either the bull is not fertile enough, there are too many cows per bull, the cows and bull are passing an infection back and forth, and/or perhaps there is a nutritional deficiency. There should be no more than about twenty-five cows per bull if you are trying to get cows bred in a tight window of time (as in a strong spring flush or in totally seasonal situations). It is fairly easy to tell if an infection is the reason; discharge will be visible on the cows' tails, or a reproductive examination will turn up evidence of a slight increase in the size of a few cows' uterine horns. Depending on when they were checked for pregnancy, a slightly increased uterine horn size may also indicate a pregnancy that is now being resorbed (early embryonic death). Bull breeding soundness exams can be conducted but require some specialized equipment to collect and analyze fresh semen at the farm. If you're considering a bull breeding soundness exam, it should be done before the breeding season starts rather than after a few miserable herd checks.

Cysts

As cows' reproductive systems "kick in" again with cooler autumn weather, they may experience cystic ovaries. Cysts can really be bothersome and generally occur when the cows rebound after a stress—this can be when cows that were skinny while at peak milk production begin putting on good condition again or after a hot spell. Cysts are traditionally treated by an injection of Cystorelin (gonadorelin-releasing hormone, which is not allowed in organic production). However, they often can be gently ruptured ("popped"). Some people would argue that rupturing a cyst can cause scarring of the ovary and hinder future fertility. I have never seen that to be the case—cows will breed back, calve in, and breed yet again. Hemorrhage of the ovary is possible with removal of a cyst, but applying some pressure for a few moments after rupturing the cyst minimizes that possibility. Definitely have a veterinarian do such a procedure.

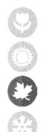

As far as natural treatments go, I've seen homeopathic *Apis mellifica* followed by *Natrum muriaticum* work consistently well for right-sided cysts, and homeopathic *Lachesis muta* followed by *Natrum muriaticum* works well on left-sided cysts. The reasoning behind the difference takes into account the differences observed experientially by persons who have been part of earlier homeopathic provings that help to describe how and why certain remedies are used. When cysts are on both ovaries, I'll use *Apis mellifica*. The standard dose of homeopathic pellets (size #40) for adult cattle is ten pellets of *Apis mellifica* or *Lachesis muta* twice daily for five days, then ten pellets of *Natrum muriaticum* twice daily for three days (basically at milking times). Breed whenever you detect a heat, no matter how minor.

Also effective for cysts (for those who don't want to use homeopathy) is HeatSeek, which is a combination plant-based remedy I developed based on a human supplement. It is given every day for six days or until heat, whichever is first. If the cow shows a heat before the twelve days of treatment are finished, simply stop treatment and breed. Another option that works is acupuncture (using injections of vitamin B_{12}) performed between the cow's short ribs on the side with the cyst. Breed whenever a heat is detectable to any degree.

Irregular Heat Cycles

Irregular heat cycles can indicate that a herd is experiencing an infection. Irregular heats or abortions in the first three to four months of pregnancy can mean bovine viral diarrhea (BVD) is in the herd. Abortions at three to five months of pregnancy could be due to BVD or leptospirosis, and abortions at six to eight months of pregnancy usually point to *Neospora caninum*.

BVD is an especially troublesome character. I say this because herds that have been well-vaccinated can still be reproductively ravaged if there is a persistently infected (PI) BVD animal on the farm. A PI animal is one that is constantly shedding BVD virus to its herdmates. This is the most common form of BVD these days (as compared to the "classic" BVD outbreak with many adult cows dying). A PI animal becomes infected when it is still in the womb, due to the pregnant cow coming into contact with BVD. The forming calf, especially if exposed to BVD between days 50–120 of pregnancy, is developing its immune system and recognizes the BVD as part of itself instead of something to react against. In effect, the BVD sneaks into the developing calf's system. The calf either dies and is aborted, is born weak and dies soon thereafter, is a runt and is sold sometime before maturity, or actually makes it into the milking string. All the while, every sneeze, cough, urination, and manure pie of this animal contains active BVD virus particles—against which a vaccine is powerless. So in herds, vaccinated or not, that experience odd reproductive problems in the first few months of gestation, BVD should be considered and investigated with your local veterinarian.

Cows that have normal ovaries with a corpus luteum (CL) usually show a heat to a shot of prostaglandin Lutalyse (dinoprost) about eighty hours after the injection. This synthetic hormone dissolves the CL so that the awaiting follicle with its egg can start going towards ovulation with its usual signs of observable heat. It is prohibited in organic production. HeatSeek has shown great results of helping cows show heat at this point of the cycle, and this is its main use for my farmers. For a normally cycling cow that simply hasn't shown heats for a long time (even if previously given Lutalyse or the various synchronization sequences), HeatSeek often gets a cow to show a heat even before completing the prescribed six doses.

In any event, whether using injections or natural treatments to get cows to show heats, there is no guarantee they will settle. That is up to your timing for AI or your bull's best judgment.

Bulls, like cows, are also affected by a hot spell. Studies have shown that bulls experiencing a body temperature of 105°F for a few days in a row will have damaged sperm. It takes a bull about forty-five days to regenerate fertile sperm, so a hot spell can really knock both bull-bred and AI herds just simply due to the hot weather.

If breeding with a bull, do try to have him run with the herd if all the safety issues of a free-running bull can be met. Having a bull run with the herd decreases your time and energy spent trying to watch cows come into heat. The bull automatically does that. If you bring

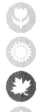

the cows to a bull in the bullpen, you still need to watch for heats, and you might as well use AI to get better genetic variety. A bull can pass an infection throughout the herd (whether in the bullpen or running with the herd). There's nothing worse for reproduction than an infected or infertile bull if a bull is all you use. Also, you will need two to three bulls if you are trying to breed your whole herd in a small period of time.

Nutritional Deficiencies

Nutritional deficiencies probably revolve more around micronutrient minerals than protein or energy, although poor energy intake will definitely hinder conception. Poor energy intake is usually obvious by seeing skinny cows for months on end. This may be seen on grazing farms when not enough effective fiber is being fed, or the fresh grass is exiting the digestive tract too quickly and cows have too loose manure (diarrhea) for too long. Keep in mind that if you spot skinny cows, there will likely be micronutrient deficiencies as well. The animals are depleting their mineral stores from their bones (the skeleton is the major bank of minerals in the body). An obvious symptom of mineral imbalance is when animals licking the soil, stones, concrete, or walls in attempts to regain minerals not available in their feed.

Some of the important microminerals include selenium, zinc, copper, manganese, and cobalt. Selenium deficiency is classically seen in newborn calves with white muscle disease; however, it is more often seen as retained placentas without a problem calving (i.e., no twins, not early, not a hard calving). Selenium also helps the immune system and can help if high somatic cell counts are a problem.

Zinc deficiency may show in reduced conception rates, increased retained placentas, hoof problems (strawberry heel, laminitis, heel cracks), low-quality milk due to high somatic cell count, and slow wound healing.

Copper deficiency may show reduced conception although heats are being seen, early embryonic death (although BVD can certainly cause early embryonic death as well), possible increase in retained placenta, and diarrhea.

Manganese deficiency may be seen as no heats or silent heats, reduced conception rate, slow or delayed ovulation, and increased abortion (although BVD, lepto, and neospora may also cause abortions).

A deficiency of cobalt, which is required for production of vitamin B_{12}, may result in reduced fertility but is more associated with increased early calf mortality.

Deficiencies of any of these micronutrients can cause an animal, especially a younger one, to have a poor hair coat and poor growth of the skeleton, legs, and joints (although parasitism can also cause symptoms of animals looking rough and not thriving). Chronically loose manure (diarrhea) will certainly deplete the animal's system of minerals as well as protein, and in adults we usually think of Johne's disease or inadequate dry hay being fed. Either way, minerals are being wasted.

Obviously, your nutritionist will be able to advise you on the proper levels of the micronutrients to feed based on what is being provided by your forages. Please keep in mind that most minerals are absorbed better through the digestive tract than by syringe and needle. Generally speaking, if the animals in your herd look sleek, have shiny hair coats, and are in proper body condition for their stage of lactation, they will most likely be able to get bred back in the time period that you would like. In short, doing your part in watching for heats, breeding them in time, feeding them well, and doing regularly scheduled reproductive examinations will enable your cows to freshen according to your schedule.

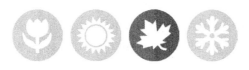

CHAPTER 14

Fresh Air and Exercise in Autumn and Winter

The seasons are changing once again, and it's time to start thinking about getting animals ready to come inside. But which animals are we talking about? Certainly the milking cows will be in more as we tend to give them the most attention. But what about the young stock? Often times we let the bred heifers stay outside with a place for them to bed down and be out of the elements and that's good. But how about the younger heifers? Oftentimes people want to bring them back inside after the grazing season just to have them under close control. But not all animals do best indoors, depending on the group of animals being considered. Why is this? Mainly because the fresh air they have been getting is so much better for them than stale barn air or shared barn air with the milking herd. As a rule, I would say that young stock should not come back into the barn until they freshen since they are at risk for pneumonia if stuck inside all winter with the older animals. It gets back to the foundations of health I periodically talk about: dry bedding, fresh air, sunshine, high-forage diets, and grazing.

Obviously, grazing of any meaningful dietary intake will not be in the equation during winter time. However, grazing way into late autumn is certainly a possibility if stockpiling forage, especially with fescue since it is more palatable after a frost. Often times it is too tough for animals to eat during the summer season. However, preclipping can soften it up to make it more palatable. Preclipping is a management technique in which the pasture to be grazed is actually mowed and allowed to wilt for two to three hours prior to actually grazing it. After a frost, fescue softens up nicely as its former toughness allows it to persist well into late autumn and even for "snow grazing" when animals eat what is still green after a few inches of snow have fallen. If grazing clover and alfalfa into the autumn, be careful, as bloat potential increases markedly after a frost. Always wait two hours until after the frost is off before setting the cows out on to clover and alfalfa. In any case, once harsh winter weather comes, any real grazing of dairy cows will be lost until next spring.

So once grazing is finished, why and how would you keep animals primarily outside? Two of the other foundational pillars of health apply: Why? For fresh air. How? With dry bedding. Certainly the freshest air will be outside. Ideally, on a daily basis animals should have the choice of going outside or staying inside. Think of calves in individual hutches being seen outside their hutch on crisp winter days as well as dairy cows walking around in a barnyard, if there's good traction and no ice, on those same crisp days. The main thing you need to keep in mind for animals that live in minimal housing outside is to minimize drafts at ground level. This could mean having a three-sided structure so the animals can get into the back areas (much like individual hutches are designed), as those chilly 36°F (3°C) rains can quickly damage animals of any size or age. And of course enough dry bedding is needed so the cows retain body warmth when lying down. Feeding enough dry matter for animals to extract calories is critical to not only keep the cows warm but also for them to grow. Feeding enough can be assessed on a daily basis by looking at rumen fill.

Which groups of animals are then best suited to be outside? Pretty much all of them. However, milking cows could be the exception as they need special attention due to their metabolic demands for lactation and the fact that their teats are being wetted and dried a few times a day by prepping for milking, pre-dipping, and post-dipping. Thus chapping is a real possibility for cows put outside right after milking (as is frostbite under certain conditions). However, I also do not recommend keeping cows inside for twenty hours out of a twenty-four-hour day for a couple reasons. One is simply that they need to get fresh air into their lungs and exercise. On days when it is not muddy or icy, there is no reason at all that cows need to be kept inside. Those sunny, deep blue skies are great for them to enjoy.

By walking around outside, the animals' muscle tone will help their lymphatic systems function optimally since the lymphatic system does not have its own circulation and relies solely on muscle movement. Have you ever noticed that a fresh cow with a retained placenta does generally better during the grazing season than a cow continually tied-in and fed lots of ensiled feed during the winter? Another reason for animals to be outside is simply for them to experience a change of environment from being confined to the indoor surroundings, allowing their senses to experience what they normally would if they were in their natural state.

Okay, so that's a set of positive reasons for having animals outside rather than continually inside during the autumn and winter months. Now let's look at life lived mainly indoors. One of the most predictable things I experience every year is getting calls about coughing calves

> By walking around outside, the animals' muscle tone will help their **LYMPHATIC SYSTEMS FUNCTION OPTIMALLY** since the lymphatic system does not have its own circulation and relies solely on muscle movement.

after a spell of bad weather in October or November. Why do calves seem to so easily start coughing when brought inside? Or similarly, why do fresh heifers sometimes break with pneumonia? Well, after enjoying fresh air since being born on pasture in the spring and perhaps having never even been inside at all yet in life, a box pen full of animals grouped together without good fresh air almost guarantees stress, thus negatively affecting the immune system. If bedding is not added or changed often enough, the dampness will compound the situation. Contact with damp concrete is the worst situation.

If young stock are also harboring stomach worms that have been accumulating all summer long while they have been on pasture, you have a recipe for disaster. This is because the calves will already be anemic from the bloodsucking internal parasites and their immune systems will be on very shaky ground. Even if the calves aren't infested but simply haven't grown well outside due to "lack of groceries," they can still easily succumb to situations of damp, stale air. (Poorly fed calves and parasitized calves are difficult to distinguish from each other.) Either way, the stresses of damp, stale air all of a sudden often overwhelms them. This is especially true in wooden and cinder block group structures. Curtain structures provide much better air movement, but always keep in mind to avoid drafts at ground level. If you do see some coughing starting, *put the animals immediately back outside* and the coughing will usually go away quickly. You might also try giving an intranasal vaccine (InForce 3) to animals to give their immune system an extra boost against specific germs *prior to coming inside*. Definitely get young stock checked or treated effectively for worms if they have been on the same small area all summer long. And remember that calves housed indoors near older animals will more likely be affected by the exhaled air of the older animals. While older animals normally have antibodies to the typical respiratory bugs, the young animals don't—and can quickly show it by starting to cough.

Simply put, animals thrive on fresh air and lose out with stale air. Except for lactating cows needing to be fed properly for production, cattle do fine outside. For their own good, we need to have them outside as much as possible (within reason) when autumn and winter weather is pleasant. This will ensure healthy lungs as well as animals happily in contact with their natural environment. Giving them daily the *choice* to be inside or outside is ideal.

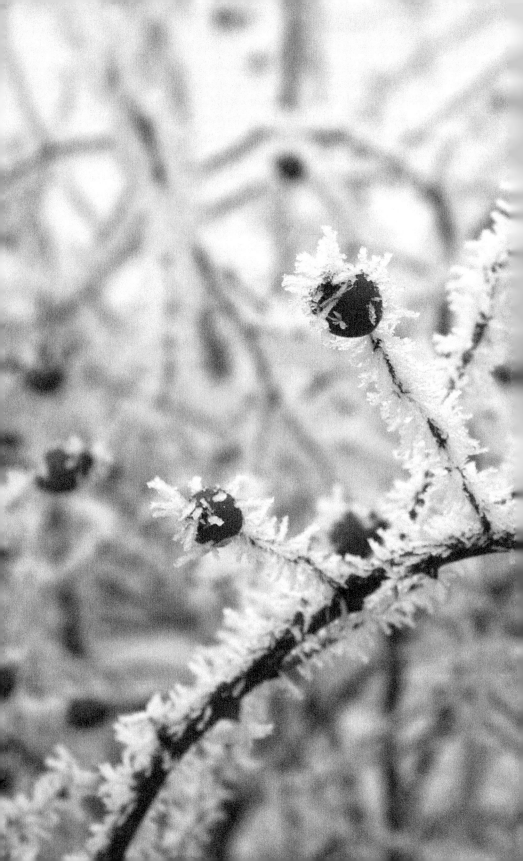

PART IV
Winter

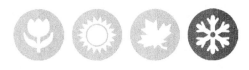

CHAPTER 15

Coughing Cows and Pneumonia

G ot anything for coughing calves? This question seems to start up again every year around late autumn and early winter—or anytime we have freezing nights and above-freezing days. With all the variable weather of winter, alternating between rain, sharp winds, and chillier temperatures, it's wise to keep an eye out for an increase in pneumonia each year. It certainly does seem to be a seasonal illness, ushered in by the changing weather and winds. Germs seem to be waiting on the walls in the barn to jump off and into the calves when the temperatures get above freezing . . . and when there is not much air movement . . . and when the bedding might be a tad soggy or damp. Though any one of these situations won't necessarily make for coughing calves, all three of these triggers acting together will almost certainly cause problems. Once you need to reach for treatments you've already lost the battle to some extent, but treating your animals in time can prevent the situation from turning into a complete train wreck, as coughing animals and full-blown pneumonia is likely to become.

The Immune System

Let's first look at the building blocks of the immune system: energy, antioxidants, vitamins, minerals, and proteins. Proper nutrition is critical. In the wintertime, however, cows will take in fewer vitamins because the vitamin content of stored feed is less than that of fresh green pasture. While healthy cows do make their own vitamins in the rumen, young stock whose rumen function is just starting may not achieve appropriate levels. Any ketotic (low-energy) animal will also not have an intact immune system. Basically any animal not eating enough feed will lack the nutrition to make enough vitamins on its own, so supplementing vitamins like A, D, and E would help boost the immune system. Vitamin E is a powerful antioxidant that helps the cells of the immune system function better. A dose of MuSe at 1cc per two hundred pounds (1cc/90kg) will boost the immune system. Being fat soluble, one shot will last for a few weeks. Vitamin C is also an antioxidant, and a dose of 5cc per hundred pounds (5cc/45kg) under the skin or in the muscle is good, but don't inject more than 30cc into one site as larger doses tend to cause abscesses (counterproductive!). Vitamin C is quickly excreted in the urine, so it can be injected daily for three days in a row. ImmunoBoost is a great non-specific immune stimulant, as it increases various forms of interferon within a couple hours after injection. It is given at the rate of 1cc per two hundred pounds (1cc/45kg) under the skin, in the muscle, or intravenously. MultiMin for trace minerals can also be given. All these angles of supplementing the animal will help to ensure a proper functioning immune system.

Consider the role of the immune system in combating disease. In the course of a respiratory challenge, if the animal is immunocompetent but has never been previously challenged by the bad bugs, it takes about ten days for the animal's own antibodies to rally and start fighting off the bad bacteria to restore equilibrium. In the first few days, during initial activation of the immune system, the animal's interferon levels increase. Interferons are proteins the body produces in response to an invading pathogen. Immune system cells, having a kind of radar, are drawn to the sites of infection. These cells (macrophages and neutrophils) kill anything that shouldn't be there. During battle, these cells are sending signals via lymphatic drainage to nearby lymph nodes. When the macrophages and neutrophils have become exhausted from the battle, you will start to see yellowish snot—that's their remains, along with dead bacteria. Other cells (lymphocytes) have been signaled and quickly mature in the nearby lymph nodes, and these cells create antibodies. Once formed, antibodies are very efficient in killing specific bacteria—antibodies seek them out, lock onto them, and destroy them quickly in expert fashion. It takes anywhere from five to ten days for lymphocytes to make antibodies to combat the invading pathogen.

Wouldn't it be great to have highly efficient antibodies already waiting to go at the first hint of a challenge? After all, every day that the damage proceeds from the bad bacteria in pneumonia means much less chance for recovery, which can quickly lead to permanent lung damage or death. The best way to have antibodies already present and functional is by vaccination (artificially induced prior exposure). *If you're going to vaccinate for only one common infectious disease on a farm, pneumonia would be it.* The intranasal vaccines (i.e. InForce 3) are easy to use and soon effective, providing quick protection by stimulating interferon production along the respiratory lining. Simply mix the dry and liquid parts together, hold the animal's head up slightly, and squirt 1cc into each nostril. This can be done for any animal at any age, even pregnant cows. If you're paranoid about vaccinating, the intranasal vaccine cannot reproduce itself in the body. The intranasal vaccine is also the only vaccine that can be given in the face of an outbreak. Never give injectable vaccines to animals showing symptoms or with fever.

Causes of Pneumonia

Pneumonia is an infection of the lungs that causes various levels of respiratory problems by impairing the lung tissue's ability to take up oxygen. Various issues can lead to pneumonia, such as primary viral infection with secondary bacterial infection, drenching cows wrong by getting liquid into the windpipe and into the lungs, and dusts and chemical vapors irritating the respiratory lining.

In a normal animal there are "good" and "bad" bacteria that line the respiratory tract, with the good keeping the bad in check when the animal is in good health. But when the animal's immune system is stressed or depressed from being outside in 35°F–40°F rain, damp/chilly air, calving time, internal parasites, stale air, damp bedding, and/or recent shipping, the normal balance can be toppled, which leads to pneumonia originating from a primary viral infection and then secondary bacterial infection, also known as enzootic calf pneumonia. This is especially likely when animals have been transported and commingled with other animals, what's known as "shipping fever." Ideally, new additions should be kept away from the herd for a couple weeks to acclimate to their new surroundings and so the herdsman can monitor them for any illness, though unfortunately this precaution is rarely observed.

Pneumonia can also strike first-calf heifers freshening in late autumn/winter and brought inside for the first time to join the milking string. Barns with poor air ventilation are the most common culprits behind this problem. Management to prevent pneumonia includes dry bedding and fresh air while avoiding drafts, as well as using one of the intranasal vaccines (TSV-2, Nasalgen, InForce 3) about a week prior to moving or mixing animals. If environmental causes like stale air, drafty air, and/or damp bedding can be corrected quickly, coughing does not necessarily proceed to pneumonia. If you can get animals that have recently started coughing outside into fresh air—if the weather is pleasant—you can stop the downward process. It's so important to not keep animals indoors all winter long. If it's a sunny, pleasant day without ice or a lot of mud, by all means put animals outside to get some fresh air and exercise. And I don't mean for only an hour. Put them out for the whole morning or afternoon, whenever possible. It will enhance their health. As most people know, it's very uncommon for calves in hutches to get respiratory problems; they can go in and out from their hutch whenever they please.

Another type of pneumonia, aspiration pneumonia, occurs when liquid gets into the lungs, most commonly when pouring a liquid into a cow's mouth (drenching). *Never* should there be liquid in the lungs. If drenching cannot be avoided entirely, it must at least be done correctly. The terrible potential effects of drenching cows incorrectly were written about in 1916 by Dr. David Roberts, a veterinarian from Wisconsin who was strongly opposed to drenching cows. It takes as little as four to eight ounces (120–240 milliliters) of liquid or gelatinous material getting into the windpipe to cause immediate and severe problems. The animal's head must be held correctly, and the farmer must pay attention. If the animal is coughing or thrashing about, she is trying to tell you something!

If you absolutely feel that you simply must drench a cow with a large amount of liquid, hold the head only very slightly above parallel to the ground, tip the bottle in, and give her a little bit. Stop and allow her to either swallow or reject it, and then repeat this process until finished. *Never* hold the animal's nose to sky, as this position will very easily allow liquids into the windpipe and lungs. (Tilting the head way back is how doctors pass a tube through the windpipe into the lungs to deliver gas anesthesia.) Giving a cow a small amount of fluid, such as an ounce (30 milliliters) a couple times a day is generally safe since it doesn't overwhelm the oral cavity all at once and spill into the windpipe like many ounces given at one time can. Ideally, farmers really should invest in a stomach tube and pump (around $100–$200) as this tool will also come in very handy when dealing with fresh cows not eating much. Five gallons of water with whatever else you would like to give (calcium, alfalfa, direct-fed microbials, botanicals, etc.) can go a long way to prevent ketosis and milk fever (low calcium). You can easily pump a cow's stomach one or two times a day for the first few days fresh if needed.

Pneumonia caused by chronic irritation of the respiratory tract by chemical vapors or dust is probably the easiest to correct—simply remove the animals from the source of irritation and put them in fresh air, and they tend to re-

> **IT TAKES AS LITTLE AS FOUR TO EIGHT OUNCES** (120–240 milliliters) of liquid or gelatinous material getting into the windpipe to cause immediate and severe problems.

cover. Typical situations that give rise to this irritation include animals housed in barns situated above a manure pit, especially during hot, humid summers with no breeze or on drizzly days in winter. The fumes from the ammonia rise and bother the animals, and they will have a dry cough until fresh breezes come by or they are moved elsewhere. If this irritation becomes long standing, it may allow true pathogens to invade the windpipe and gain access to the lower lungs. Occasionally, dust coming down from activity above the cows or from molds on barn walls can cause respiratory symptoms.

Of the three types of pneumonia mentioned, aspiration pneumonia is the hardest to deal with and often proves fatal or leaves the cow severely debilitated and non-functional. It is basic biology that we need to breathe before we do anything else, and therefore if we can't breathe we can't eat. Pneumonia due to irritation is the easiest to reverse, if the cause is recognized soon enough and the animals are removed from it. However, if not caught quickly, enough damage can be done to facilitate bacterial invasion of the lung fields, leading to bacterial pneumonia. Infectious pneumonia due to a virus or bacteria is always a concern, especially on organic farms since antibiotics can't be used without permanent removal of the animal. Therefore prevention with the intranasal vaccine is key, especially if the farm has a history of this kind of pneumonia.

Enzootic Calf Pneumonia

Let's take a closer look at that first type of pneumonia. Oftentimes I'll receive a call when a calf is sick enough that a farmer observes a change in normal behavior. Symptoms usually include a cough, nasal discharge, not coming up to eat, and perhaps a rough coat. When checking the calf in question, I usually will hear rough or raspy lung sounds of varying intensity, find a fever of typically 103.2°F–104.8°F (39.6°C–40.4°C), observe an increased respiratory rate, and hear an obvious cough. But when I'm in the pen to examine the sick calf, others will begin coughing when rustled up. Upon examining them, they will usually have milder symptoms than the sickest calf but be on the path to becoming just as sick. This condition of calves is called enzootic calf pneumonia. The sickest calf is suffering from secondary bacterial invasion of the lungs (usually due to *Mannheimia hemolytica* or *Pasteurella multocida*). The bacterial infection is secondary to a primary viral infection. The primary viral infection "punches holes" along the respiratory tract, and opportunistic bacteria that are always present colonize these holes and rapidly invade deep into the lung tissue, often creating a fatal secondary bacterial pneumonia if left untreated for too long. In general, animals can withstand viral challenges if their immune system is functioning well; that is, if they are not stressed, not parasitized, and their environment is optimal. They can benefit from vaccinating with the intranasal vaccine at that point.

My thoughts on pneumonia in cattle haven't changed much over time, although they are a bit more defined at this point. More and more, I have come to think that damp bedding is the critical factor for calves to come down with pneumonia. It certainly isn't the only factor—poor ventilation is also a main culprit, although mixing poor ventilation with damp bedding is a sure recipe for pneumonia in calves. Sometimes I place my palms upon the ground in pens with coughing calves, and the bedding is nearly always damp or worse. Young animals will never feel comfortable lying on constantly damp bedding. It just won't do. Straw and fodder are great, and sawdust can be good—these allow moisture to seep down before it accumulates at the surface where the animals are. Newspaper is not good in this regard as dampness stays right on top once it is wetted. Dry bedding is critical—how would you like it if you had damp sheets and blankets for your bedding?

The beautiful stone barns here in southeastern Pennsylvania are actually one of the main areas for pneumonia germs to lurk, it seems. When we have damp, chilly weather—as we so often do in late autumn and early winter—the old stone structures remain moist, and air does not move well, especially in corners. Those corners happen to be where calf box stalls are. The only structures worse than the old stone barns are cinder-block buildings, since they tend to be chilly in general. Dampness in block buildings is a major factor of pneumonia, especially together with damp bedding. The good thing about block buildings is that you can knock blocks out and put in curtains, which

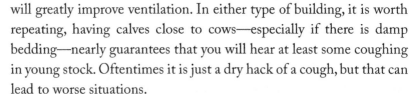

will greatly improve ventilation. In either type of building, it is worth repeating, having calves close to cows—especially if there is damp bedding—nearly guarantees that you will hear at least some coughing in young stock. Oftentimes it is just a dry hack of a cough, but that can lead to worse situations.

Another factor that can compromise the health of calves is the presence of parasites. Basically, calves that are parasitized will be more susceptible to any infection and will not have the vitality to effectively battle the germs they encounter. It is therefore important to check for obvious parasitism in calves that are coughing, especially on the organic farms where very limited use of conventional wormers is allowed on a diagnosed parasite problem (when methods acceptable to organic have not been successful). The wormers allowed are fenbendazole, moxidectin, and ivermectin. By getting rid of the parasitic worms, the animal will immediately become stronger and other treatments will be more effective.

Prevention

Of course preventing the coughs is best, but it's often difficult to do. Certainly dry bedding, fresh air, clean water, and top-notch nutrition are critical. And allowing dairy calves to nurse from their mother cows is as close to Mother Nature as can be found—actually, it *is* Mother Nature.

If you must keep calves near cows in the stable, keep only the youngest (pre-weaned) calves inside. If they are on whole milk, they will probably do fine. Then once weaned keep calves outside, especially recently weaned calves, as their immune systems take a few months to adjust to their new diet (usually poorer quality feed).

Which is worse: poor ventilation and cold, damp bedding or poor ventilation and a warm, stuffy barn? The answer, in my opinion, is that they are equally bad, but perhaps the warm, stuffy barn is worse for the just-fresh adult cows, and the cold, damp bedding and poor ventilation are worse for young stock. Good, clean, crisp air is great for any type of cattle: calves, yearlings, and cows. They are meant to be outside after all, not cooped up inside all the time. If calves must be inside in tie-stalls during the winter, have some windows open above them to allow good air flow, which will help move accumulated ammonia away from surface areas of calf pens and thereby lessen irritation of the windpipe by ammonia (from urine).

Without doubt, individual hutches are the way to go to minimize coughing and pneumonia. There are few things nicer to see than a calf chewing its cud while lying down comfortably on dry bedding inside its hutch on a cold rainy and windy day. The next best prevention of coughing calves is raising calves in a super hutch as a social group, but you need to watch out for any cross-sucking of penmates' teats. Individual hutches with an enclosed, fenced area that allow the calf to decide whether to be inside or outside are the best for respiratory health. Remember to clean and move hutches to new locations after every calf to minimize contamination between calves. Some folks in the animal science community are now raising questions about individual hutches since calves are very social creatures and like to be in groups. I say that temporarily having the youngest calves in separate hutches to prevent respiratory disease trumps grouping calves just to enable social interaction, especially if respiratory disease has been a problem on a farm. They will be grouped together fairly soon anyway, once weaned.

In more northern areas, calf jackets are an excellent item to have for any calf, especially a sick calf in the wintertime. Regular healthy calves that are outside in the wintertime need as much as a third more energy in their food rations to maintain body heat. Studies in the upper Midwest have shown that using calf jackets can reduce the need for that extra feed. If they use too many calories just to stay warm, their immune system will not be at peak performance. When a calf is sick in the winter, it is almost a basic requirement to use a jacket or blanket to keep their body heat from escaping. (This is true also for a down cow in the field in the wintertime, especially overnight or when the winds are sharp.)

The multi-calf kennels are okay if calves have the room to go outside, like the outdoor areas for hutches. Multi-calf kennels designed so that the animals cannot freely go in and out can cause problems. I find the wooden multi-calf kennels usually harbor bugs that cause digestive problems (scours) associated with coccidia at some point. Though somewhat difficult compared to individual hutches, kennel buildings can be moved, too, and really should be, at least once in a while, to avoid the typical problems with accumulating parasites.

Using box stalls to raise a group of calves in the main cow barn is risky. Box stalls in barns obviously cannot be moved, and perhaps that is part of the reason why they seem to be magnets for diseases, especially those near the adult cows. It is just difficult to clean them out very often. And if one of a group gets sick, it's more likely that others in the group will, too. If you're thinking the heat generated in a bedded pack kills germs, you're correct, at least if you're continuously adding bedding as a carbon source. I'm not sure which material is best to mix in, just as long as there is a good amount of bedding.

What to Look For

It is critical to know how the lungs sound to decide which treatment route to go. If the lungs sound raspy and rough, then natural treatment can be very effective. If you hear "wet" abscess sounds, the animal needs antibiotics. And if you hear consolidated lungs, it's too late for anything. Consolidated lungs are lungs with permanently damaged areas that are compacted and can no longer inflate. Usually the worst animal is the first to catch the farmer's attention.

Oftentimes the sickest calf in the group will already have serious lung damage (consolidation). A consolidated lung means that air entering the lungs through the windpipe never gets effectively absorbed because the areas of diseased lung tissue are no longer functional. By listening with the stethoscope, a vet can alert the farmer as to how much permanently damaged tissue there is. These calves, if they survive, usually show respiratory problems in a couple of years when heavy in calf in the hot summer days. Aggressive antibiotic and anti-inflammatory therapy is their only hope—but the permanently damaged tissue will still be useless later on. Animals simply don't function well with less than 100 percent lung capacity (neither do humans).

Other than coughing, symptoms include wet rings around the eyes, with the whites of the eyes themselves appearing slightly pink or reddened in general—this is the case when the initial virus is affecting the animal. Some animals may also show very small blisters at the bottom outside edge of the nostrils, and occasionally white plaques may be seen within the nostrils if infectious bovine rhinotracheitis (IBR) is the cause (it is rare to see such blisters or plaques). Eventually a mucopurulent discharge ("snot") will be seen from the eyes and nostrils as the bacterial stage sets in. There will typically be other animals in the group coughing, but they remain bright, alert, and keep on eating. Checking the lung sounds and temperatures is critical in order to decide how best to treat them. Within a group of animals will be a variety of temperatures, lung sounds, and displays of general illness, depending on the stress level. The worst affected are usually those recently weaned, with poor body condition, parasitized, and/or just fresh from calving. Using a stethoscope, listen for lung sounds that range from slightly raspy to harsh friction rubs, worse yet are fluid sounds/abscesses, and the worst being only windpipe sounds in certain lung areas (when areas of the lung are no longer functional). With only mild to harsh sounds, animals generally keep on eating, if the fever isn't too high. If no action is taken, each animal will become ill to various degrees, depending on how virulent the viral or bacterial strain is and how they individually react to the challenge. A cow that has severely compromised lung function will often be heard grunting with every breath, an indication that the animal will likely die within a few hours. If pneumonia is contained to the viral stage only, the situation isn't too bad; however, it almost always degenerates to the bacterial stage, which can easily lead to death if left unchecked.

Treatments

In my time practicing veterinary medicine, I have treated animals of all ages sick with pneumonia, both on organic and conventional farms. No matter which type of farm is experiencing a pneumonia outbreak, the sickest animal will usually end up having permanent lung damage since it is too far advanced in the disease process due to starting treatment too late. On farms that are not certified organic, the best and most quickly effective treatment will be an antibiotic such as ceftiofur

(Naxcel or Excenel), florfenicol (Nuflor), or tilmicosin (Micotil). Tilmicosin is very effective for calf pneumonia, as can be florfenicol, but the tilmicosin seems more effective in my experience. Naxcel works nicely, but it needs daily injecting. Alarmingly, although ceftiofur was originally designed to treat shipping fever (pneumonia), it doesn't seem to be as effective as it once was. Bacteria seem to be mounting resistance against it in barns where it is used frequently. However, if a farmer only rarely uses antibiotics on his farm, it can still work very well. Oxytetracycline (LA-200) may work, but oftentimes it only puts a damper on the pneumonia and doesn't clear the infection. I would *not* use penicillin against pneumonia. If reaching for an antibiotic, remember that antibiotics need a functioning immune system to do their job. They work by giving the immune system time to rally instead of becoming overwhelmed and beaten, which certainly can happen in pneumonia. Therefore, keep in mind injectable antioxidants like vitamins C and E. Withholding times of antibiotics and the time it takes to administer the medicine will usually dictate which of these medicines will be used. If the animal hasn't degenerated to having portions of the lung consolidated and nonfunctional, recovery is usually rapid.

Antibiotics can be excellent for bacterial pneumonia, but if an organic animal is given an antibiotic, it is banished from organic production forever (in the U.S. certified organic system). On organic farms, pneumonia treatment relies much more on non-synthetic measures, namely boosting the immune system using plant medicines with strong antibacterial effects and moving the animal to fresh air. However, according to U.S. law, organic farmers cannot withhold prohibited antibiotic treatments just to keep an animal organic. This restriction makes my life as a veterinarian more interesting and challenging, especially when faced with a disease like pneumonia that can easily kill an animal if not quickly and effectively treated.

A key point to keep in mind is that natural treatment of pneumonia using biological methods tends to take a little longer for the animals to normalize—about five to seven days instead of the one to two days with antibiotics. But then the animals have essentially healed themselves and should be stronger in the long run. My rule of thumb is to stick with the biological approach if the animal is holding its own and going the right way, but switch to antibiotics if the animal is worsening. *If treatment is started soon enough*, I have seen countless cases of pneumonia cleared up by using purely biological treatments to work with the animal's own immune system.

Early Intervention

Let's say that you have a bunch of calves inside that are obviously coughing and you decide to check their temperatures (which I would recommend doing for *any* animal that is not acting normally). If temperatures are normal (100.5°F–102.5°F) and the worst calf is eating, great. Move them to fresh air and simply keep a close eye on them. If a pen of calves coughs when they're rustled up and moving around, but they are eating, then try using high doses of garlic in the feed. The addition will make the feed tastier to them, and garlic is an excellent natural antibiotic and anti-viral. Temperatures in the 105°F–106°F range usually indicate a viral challenge to the calf, and the fever indicates that the animal is actively fighting the infection. Agri-Dynamics' Pulmonex or CowMaster Get Well are good garlic formulas.

In viral infections (as indicated by high fever), antibiotics are of no primary use. Botanical or homeopathic remedies like aconite (recent onset) and belladonna (fever with throbbing heartbeat, reddish-pink dry mouth, dilated pupils) are more in order. Wet coughs indicate that you should use Antimonium tart, if it's early in the infection. Immune-boosting substances would be very valuable in this case. If the animal is bright, alert, and eating, do not necessarily try to drop the fever with aspirin and flunixin (both are on the National List of Allowed Synthetics for Livestock*). However, if the animal is droopy and not eating, dropping the fever will benefit the patient by making it feel well enough to start eating and taking in nutrients so that it can fend off the infection better in general if possible.

If the calves cough when rustled up and have a slight fever (102.6°F–103.2°F), they need treatment—do not take the "let's wait

---

* 7CFR205.603

and see" approach. They're bound to get worse in my experience. I would start right away with natural products that enhance the immune system. The quickest and most effective would be to use pre-formed antibodies that will neutralize the bad bacteria and their associated toxins. My original success in treating pneumonia without antibiotics was during a rip-roaring shipping fever outbreak on an organic farm that had recently been assembled. The commercial product called Bovi-Sera (also known as multi-serum) worked quickly. It can be injected under the skin or in the muscle or given intravenously. The antibodies and antitoxins will remain effective for about ten to twelve days, giving the animal's immune system much-needed time to clear the germs causing the infection on its own. ImmunoBoost stimulates interferon production, which helps the animal from a slightly different angle. While both products augment the animal's natural immune system, the antibodies (IgG) work against specific bacteria that are the cause of the problem while the interferon stimulates the non-specific arm of the immune system (natural killer cells). Giving a one-time treatment of each of these products is all that is needed as far as injections. Following up by giving oral herbal tinctures is a smart way to add healing power.

> **MANY PEOPLE LIKE TO USE HOMEOPATHIC REMEDIES,** which is what I got my start with as a herdsman. Homeopathy holds a special place in my heart, but it does take determination to figure out which exact remedies to use for the specific symptoms of each individual animal.

An herbal product I have developed called Get Well (and Agri-Dynamics' Phyto-Biotic) is a very strong combination of antibacterial herbal components, namely garlic, goldenseal, barberry, and ginseng. This natural antibiotic formula, if used on its own, is only for moderately affected animals—not severely affected ones that are also not eating well. To treat an adult cow, add 90cc Get Well/Phyto-Biotic to a 500cc bottle of dextrose (essentially topping off a brand new dextrose bottle) and give it in the vein to achieve very high circulating levels of antibacterial effects. I usually do the following treatment when called to treat a cow that has pneumonia (or hot coliform mastitis): I start the intravenous treatment first with the bottle of dextrose and 90cc Get Well/Phyto-Biotic. Then I run in 250cc Bovi-Sera or multi-serum antibodies along with 5cc ImmunoBoost mixed into that and finish the treatment with 250cc–500cc vitamin C. Since giving an IV to a small calf is difficult, it's also a good idea to give 5cc–10cc each of vitamin C and vitamin B-complex in the back leg muscle once daily for four to five days, as well as a dose of vitamin E and selenium (MuSe). Multi-Min for tracemineral support is good also.

For dosing young pre-weaned calves, administer 5cc of the Get Well/Phyto-Biotic by mouth twice daily for four to five days. It can be put into the milk. For weaned calves, use 5cc–8cc each dose. You will need to catch up each calf twice daily for four to five days to administer this treatment, but many people don't mind, due to the positive results.

For individual calves needing an extra boost, use of an injectable colostrum-whey product like Agri-Dynamics' Biocel-CBT is handy. Biocel-CBT is a biologic derived from colostrum-whey and is a source of some general immune-enhancing compounds that can help a calf get over a mild respiratory infection on its own without using antibiotics. Give calves 5cc under the skin once daily for three days. It can also be used in adult cows as well at the rate of 35cc under the skin once daily for three days.

Many people like to use homeopathic remedies, which is what I got my start with as a herdsman. Homeopathy holds a special place in my heart, but it does take determination to figure out which exact remedies to use for the specific symptoms of each individual animal. However, there are some remedies that seem to be generally indicated for coughing calves: Antimonium tart 30C for wet coughs, Bryonia 30C for dry coughs, Aconite 30C for the earliest signs (but not if they've broken a sweat), and a combination of Bryonia/Urtica/Belladonna 200C for general fever and respiratory involvement. For calves, five pellets two to four times daily is the usual dose. In homeopathy, it is critical to change remedies as symptoms change. And unlike antibiotics, which require the animal to complete the full course of treatment, homeopathics can be stopped at any time that there is no longer a problem. The key is to *not* keep giving the same homeopathic on and on if the symptoms are changing and/or worsening.

These natural treatments have been successful in all but the worst cases, which can still be treated with a conventional antibiotic in a day or two if the animals are not yet displaying signs of consolidated lung (open-mouth breathing and standing with a straightened neck). Yes, natural treatments are labor intensive, but that is sometimes the trade-off when not relying on antibiotic treatments. One thing to point out is that if an animal has a second serious problem at the same time while having pneumonia (bad uterus/metritis or parasitized) and is depressed, go directly to the conventional antibiotic route. In these cases the animal is so low in vitality that it simply cannot stave off an attack on two fronts without seriously strong measures. However, for any group of animals eating well, with a very slight, light, dry cough, using natural treatments and good management (fresh air and dry bedding) can work quite well.

During one winter, out of roughly one hundred animals on five separate organic farms treated with natural means, we only reverted to conventional antibiotics on four animals (two heifers and two cows). Two other cows died using natural treatments (both fresh and one had a bad uterus also). In the days before modern antibiotics, pneumonia killed or left many animals useless. By using a *multipronged* approach with natural treatments, the results are not too far different than with antibiotics. The key is to jump on the problem quickly before irreversible changes take place.

Conclusion

I have spent a lot of time talking about pneumonia. Why? Because pneumonia is to be avoided at all costs—especially on organic farms where quickly reaching for an antibiotic is simply not an everyday option. I have covered various angles of pneumonia—the kinds, the causes, the prevention, and the treatment. To put it simply, pneumonia can easily be prevented and management should definitely strive to do so. Keeping in mind the building blocks of the immune system and the challenges to the animals from their environment is critical. If pneumonia does occur, initiating natural treatment without delay can result in very favorable outcomes. Natural treatments work by stimulating, augmenting and strengthening the animal's own immune system. And, depending on a farm's history with pneumonia, vaccinating with an intranasal vaccine in a timely manner is very effective at preventing what could otherwise be a hard battle against pneumonia in the barn.

Remember that the USDA National Organic Program requires animals to be given appropriate treatments for their diagnosed condition in order to restore them to health. Withholding appropriate treatment just to keep the animal organic is illegal and grounds for decertification. Unfortunately, when an animal has been given a prohibited material like an antibiotic, it must be removed from the herd. But most rational farmers would rather see an animal saved by an antibiotic than have a dead organic animal, especially when considering the good prices for replacement animals on the open market. And besides, most farmers sell a few animals a year anyway, so animals successfully treated in time by antibiotics can go live on a different farm.

On organic farms, we need to assess if the animal is showing signs of mild, moderate, or severe lung disease. If there is only mild or moderate disease, the general idea is to stimulate and aid the immune system to support the animal so it can recover. If the lungs sound dry but raspy or harsh (basically functional) and are moving air when listening by stethoscope, the non-antibiotic approach can work well. If the animal is coughing and has an increased respiratory rate along with shallow breathing, and there is congestion and "wet" abscess sounds when listening with a stethoscope, and the animal is running a high fever (103.6°F–105.4°F), she will need an antibiotic. Do not delay.

The described treatments for pneumonia that I recommend are based on my direct clinical experience. However, without a doubt, especially in pneumonia, an ounce of prevention is worth a pound of cure. Remember, fresh air and dry bedding are basic safeguards for animals against changes in the weather.

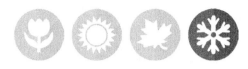

CHAPTER 16

Dry Cow Care

In general there are three parts to dry cow management: the time period of drying off, the dry period itself, and then just before the cow calves. Drying off cows often happens during winter in anticipation of spring calving.

Time to Go Dry

First, we need to start with drying off the cow. Our major goals are to make sure that her immune system is functioning well and that the udder stops milk production. We can best help the immune system by feeding the cow correctly. The cow's nutritional needs are most easily observed by its body condition. At dry-off, a cow's body condition score should ideally be between 3.5–4 (1 being skinny, 5 being fat). She ought to be in positive energy balance, having gained weight since peak lactation months before and yet not too fat. If over-conditioned at dry-off, do not stuff her full of corn silage during the dry period as that will fatten her up worse yet. I guess I'd rather see a slightly overweight cow going dry than a skinny cow going dry; the rapidly growing calf will keep taking energy from the skinny cow, thereby leaving the skinny cow's immune system functioning poorly. The dry period is *not* the time to put weight onto a cow, as fat gained at this time then may clog the liver and reduce its vital functions.

Why do we need the immune system to function during the dry period? I think the answer is rather clear—to have a "well" cow—but also we need to consider that the cow will not be looked after as closely as her lactating herd mates. She therefore needs to rely on herself a bit more during periods of high stress (like extreme cold weather). We need to have the cow's udder happy and quiet, and that requires a healthy immune system as well as clean, comfortable surroundings.

Drying off cows can be stressful for a cow, simply due to changing its daily routine of milking twice a day. The more they are still milking, the harder it can be for cows to switch into dry mode. Cows can easily be dried off when making less than 20 pounds of milk a day. If still producing higher amounts of milk, simply give them poor feed-quality roughage—even straw—for a few days to dramatically cut milk production.

For normal cows, it is well known that completely stopping milking is better than milking a cow once a day for a few days, then every other day for a few days, and then drying off. The reason for completely stopping milking at one time is that the cow's hormones will respond the best; the cow's brain will get the signal that it is time to stop producing milk. Do not milk her for five days. If the udder is touched during that time it will signal the cow to continue producing milk. You should dip the cow's teats twice daily for two weeks, *after the initial five-day dry-off*, while the natural keratin plugs that keep out environmental bugs becomes fully functional. Many teat dips used in conventional farming are also allowed in organic farming, especially those with iodine or hydrogen peroxide as the active ingredient (but check with an organic certifier first). In the conventional world, there is a handy commercial teat plug made of sodium subnitrite (Orbeseal) that many use. While this product is okay for organic use in Canada and the European Union, it is not approved for U.S. organic use, unfortunately. We thus need to let the natural plug form as fast as possible, so don't touch the udder because oxytocin will be released from the brain to let down the residual milk in the udder and she will drip, inviting germs from the environment into the teat.

While drying off can be a stressful period for the cow, it is only very temporary and not at all like the stresses associated with calving time. Most farmers plan for a traditional sixty-day dry period. I support this. There are studies of cows dried off for only thirty to forty-five days, but the results are mixed as far as cow health is concerned. At dry-off, most cows will have been declining in milk to a point where not milking them will not cause any major problems, other than the cows' temporary discomfort of an udder not being milked out any longer.

The dry period is a time when the udder is "on vacation" and can rest prior to resuming milk production the next lactation. During its resting time, many problems can be cleaned up by the cow herself if her immune system is working well. But sometimes we may sleep better if we administer a treatment to a cow that has had some problems in the past.

What about cows that have high somatic cell counts? In a very conservative sense, any cow above 200,000 somatic cell count (SCC) could be considered a high-count cow. But in reality, I would say that it depends on the trend of the cow over lactation. If she has been at 400,000 (linear score of five) the whole lactation, I wouldn't necessarily treat her with anything unless she is showing some flakes at dry-off. Cows at 800,000 (linear score of six) need extra attention at dry-off, especially cows that may have been very low during most of the lactation but have quickly increased near dry-off. While it is normal for cows to have a higher SCC toward dry-off, obvious increases in SCC or flakes demand extra attention. Cows with linear SCC of seven, eight, or nine definitely need some kind of treatment so they don't flare up during the dry period. Treatments to dry off cows may range from some extra nutritional components all the way to injectables and udder infusions.

If you have a cow to dry off and she has some slight mastitis (high CMT or slight flakes and minor swelling), I would strongly suggest using a colostrum-whey product, like Biocel-CBT from Agri-Dynamics or Phyto-Mast, a botanical product infused into the teats that have anti-bacterial healing properties. Or, if it is just a high somatic cell count on the California Mastitis Test (CMT) or Dairy Herd Improvement Association (DHIA), using ImmunoBoost can help lower the SCC for a couple months—just the right length of time for the dry period. If you're interested in using homeopathic remedies, ten pellets of silicea 30C can be given orally or in the vulva once weekly for the duration of the dry period. This may help soften any firmness of the quarter and stimulate the cow to deal with any chronic mastitis.

In the case of problem cows that have had high somatic cell counts or actual mastitis at the time of dry-off, we do need to milk them a little longer than planned, using natural antibacterial treatments to cleanse the local area and/or stimulate the immune system to overcome the current problem. Phyto-Mast has been shown in a study at North Carolina State University to significantly help with problematic milk quality at dry-off compared to nothing at all. For simple high somatic cell count, ImmunoBoost is good for stimulating the general immune system before dry-off and should be given two to three days prior. Both of these treatments are okay for use in organic.

What is a healthy udder? For dry-off purposes it can be said that cows that have a linear somatic cell count of zero to four (less than 200,000 SCC) are in fine shape. These really, truly don't need any kind of dry-off therapy (tubes or shots), whether conventional or organic.

If coliform mastitis has happened in more than one dry or fresh cow within a thirty- to forty-cow herd during the previous year, consider using a coliform vaccine like J-5 to prevent this very damaging condition. Vaccinating a herd of forty to fifty cows against coliform is cheaper than one clinical case (direct treatment costs for the sick cow and recuperation time, loss of milk, and possible loss of a quarter). Most coliform cases happen either in the first two weeks dry or in the last two weeks prior to freshening when the natural teat plugs haven't yet formed or are dissolving prior to lactation, respectively. It also occurs in fresh cows that leak milk, especially when there is sawdust or ground peanut hull bedding. Dipping teats twice daily may help.

The dual purpose Phyto-Mast botanical mastitis tubes are clinically proven in studies to enhance milk quality in cows naturally infected by environmental strep and environmental staph during lactation and at dry-off. It helps moderately swollen quarters and quarters with actual flakes or stringy mastitis. Many farmers say that cows often times come back into lactation better than they did the previous year. I would recommend Phyto-Mast for drying off cows that have a linear SCC of seven, eight, and nine or if their SCC has jumped up recently just prior to dry-off. The usual treatment is to use one tube in each of the cow's quarters and then dry her off. A minor variation on this would be to use the tubes and then wait five days, check the cow's milk, and re-treat if needed.

Most farmers use these Phyto-Mast tubes for cows mainly during lactation. Phyto-Mast has been allowed by various organic certifiers across the country. The normal treatment for lactating cows is two tubes in the affected quarter for two milkings in a row, holding the bad quarter out of the tank during treatment and for twelve hours extra. Using a quarter milker for any quarters selected to not go into the bulk tank is recommended to avoid any aroma in the tank.

Dried-Off

After two weeks of being dry, problems are usually minimal with dry cows.

In general, dry cows should be monitored twice daily, especially for irregular swelling of the udders during the first two weeks and last two weeks of their dry period. In the middle of the dry period, monitoring dry cows for feed intake is crucial. Any dry cow not eating normally or showing any significant body condition changes should be pulled aside for closer inspection. If a cow is not eating well while heavily pregnant, the calf becomes a parasite (in a sense) and its needs will be met first, drawing down the mother animal even more. If the dry cow becomes ke-

> **MOST COLIFORM CASES** happen either in the first two weeks dry or in the last two weeks prior to freshening when the natural teat plugs haven't yet formed or are dissolving prior to lactation, respectively.

totic because it lacks sufficient energy intake for its needs, its immune system will suffer and opportunistic infections could strike. Also, any discharge from the vulva (aside from normal straw-colored mucus) should have you examining the cow. Any red-colored discharge from a pregnant cow, especially a cow further along in pregnancy, means that the reproductive tract must be checked. A red discharge is a red flag.

Unfortunately, usually during summertime field work, dry cows are not usually as closely monitored. If a problem is allowed time to fester, the then seriously sick and heavily pregnant cow will need quick and effective treatment. For example, a cow that gets mastitis in the middle of the dry period will oftentimes develop a very hard quarter with a stinking, pudding-like discharge and a significant fever. If it's not noticed right away, the mastitis can become life threatening and the cow might abort the calf. As the udder becomes very tight with the mastitis building up inside, circulation to the udder will become impaired, and then, occasionally, gangrene mastitis will develop. This is a disaster, and I've only ever seen antibiotics effectively save the life of the cow (and calf). Sometimes, a farmer will notice a cow with a hard quarter, but she is eating well and looks quite healthy. Although it is too late to save the quarter from whatever bacteria invaded the gland, be thankful that the cow made it through the active infection without your help.

Pre-fresh

Ideally, any springing heifer or cow should be on the farm where she will calve at least three weeks prior to calving so the mother cow will be exposed to the germs at the farm and create colostrum with the appropriate antibodies. Due to the placental barriers between the cow and the calf, calves are born with no antibodies and need one gallon of colostrum within the first six to twelve hours of life for maximal antibody absorption from the colostrum. The calf will then be protected against the environmental bugs it will face in its first couple months of life. Any vaccinations you want to do need to be done at about three weeks prior to the anticipated calving date in order to the colostrum enough time to become enriched. The only exception would be the intranasal vaccine to help guard against pneumonia of first-calf heifers coming fresh into the barn during the winter time. Some typical vaccinations would be against coliform mastitis (J-5), which cows can easily get on some farms around freshening time, as well as the rota/corona viruses that can cause diarrhea in calves. Scour Guard 4KC is my vaccine of choice against calf diarrhea, uterine infection, and coliform mastitis. It is pretty much useless to vaccinate cows between two weeks before and two weeks after freshening since their immune system is suppressed due to the release of internal hormones associated with the end of pregnancy and beginning of lactation. If it is the cow's very first time vaccinating with the Scour Guard 4KC, you'll need to vaccinate twice (three to four weeks apart). The best time would be about a week prior to dry-off and then again about a month prior to calving date.

If a farm is having problems with retained placentas when there are no calving difficulties, then there may be a selenium deficiency in the dry cow ration. To best prevent retained placentas (and all the problems that go with them), give an injection of MuSe at two weeks prior to calving. The combination of vitamin E and selenium is a fat-soluble complex and will give good levels for about three weeks. This can also help ovarian/egg health in the upcoming lactation. Giving 10cc MuSe under the skin or in the muscle would be a good idea prior to dry-off but especially once the cow is dry and ready to calve in about two weeks. Giving MuSe at this time will also help reduce high SCC coming into lactation. Alternatively, if a farmer does not want to give injections, feeding Sel-Plex daily to the dry cows could be beneficial. Sel-Plex contains an organically bound selenium source that is very bio-available to the cow from her gut. However, the sodium selenite that is found in MuSe is the form of selenium taken up by the ovarian cells.

Additionally, during the last two weeks before freshening, daily administration of ten pellets of homeopathic caulophyllum 30C is thought to help to prepare the uterus for calving. To help actual contractions during labor, switch to the botanical tincture of caulophyllum (blue cohosh) using ten drops every twenty minutes, as some European studies have shown this to have positive effects on the muscles of the uterus.

If milk fever is an issue on the farm at freshening, try giving two ounces of apple cider vinegar two times daily for two weeks prior to freshening ("2-2-2"). For reasons not too well understood, this simple treatment works wonderfully in preventing milk fever most of the time. I have gotten only positive feedback from farmers when they have started this prevention program. The apple cider vinegar can be easily hidden in ensiled feeds. For organic farms, the apple cider vinegar need not be organic if feeding only for those two weeks. If you continue feeding it on and on into lactation to help increase butterfat, it has to be certified organic. But routinely feeding vinegar seems to diminish the milk fever preventive effect.

If you know your cow is carrying twins (usually detected by ultrasound), dry her off seven to ten days earlier than normal, as cows with twins will calve seven to ten days sooner than the expected due date. Closely watching dry cows within two weeks of the due date is very important because the teat plug starts dissolving and there is an increased likelihood of environmental mastitis. This may be even more likely in older cows a day or two before freshening if they are starting to be low in calcium (subclinical milk fever) as all muscles, including teat sphincters, are weakened and may be more open to the environment than they should be. Dip the teats twice daily for those last two weeks, and if she is really bagged up, go ahead and pre-milk her so she doesn't become a "leaker." But beware that her colostrum may not be as high quality for the calf.

Exercise is critical for dry cows, and they should get plenty of it during their "vacation" time. It strengthens all muscles, including the uterine muscles needed for calving. Exercise will also help move lymphatic drainage away from the udder while it is refreshing itself and keep cows from getting fat. Clean, grassy pasture helps udders stay clean, and time on pasture has also been shown to help hoof health. The most natural place for a cow to calve is on pasture when the weather is nice. Walking to check on dry cows on pasture will also keep you in good shape!

Loving a Cow to Death

After twenty years now in practice and trying to sort through cases that are presented, there is one kind of case that particularly sticks out in my mind—that of "loving a cow to death." Now what on earth could I mean by that? Well, let's back up a moment and think about our animals and how they normally live. What is their normal response and reaction to their immediate surroundings and life events in general? For example, if a cow just calves, what is she normally like? Typically, a cow will go off feed about twelve to twenty-four hours prior to calving as internal changes rapidly progress—uterine contractions become stronger and stronger until actual birthing takes place. What is a cow's normal response to having just given birth? Basically to rest and take care of the calf. They should also pass the placenta within about six hours of calving. Offering them water and hay are basics that a farmer needs to do at minimum as well as making sure the calf is sucking on the cow for its colostrum or gets enough colostrum via stomach tube. Some farmers, out of true care and concern, will go the extra step and "help" the cow even though she truly doesn't need it, and this can lead to real problems. For instance, if a cow cleans (passes the placenta), there is absolutely no need to put anything into the uterus "to help her along." Apparently some salesmen tell farmers to put a certain kind of bolus into the uterus, even if she cleaned normally. Wrong thing to do! Why fix something if it isn't broken? Or, if a cow is a little slow a day after calving, many people like to give a pill of one sort or another to a cow to help jump-start the rumen, even though she is eating (just too slowly for the likes of the farmer). Unfortunately, pill gun injuries happen, which means the pill gun itself damages the mouth or throat lining and ends up causing a raging infection. These are very bad and usually don't cure without using an antibiotic because of the ever-present oral bacteria that continually infect and reinfect the injury site. Or, more commonly, people like to drench a cow with a liquid of some sort to help the cow get eating better or to help her immune system, because she is "a little slow." You don't know how many cows I have checked for being "off-feed" when just fresh and then I find that the lungs are damaged due to drenching the cow inappropriately. This is nearly impossible to correct, even with the strongest antibiotics, since no fluids should ever be in the lungs in the first place. The most offending products are the calcium products for low-calcium conditions—they really burn the lung tissue intensely.

Worse is when an older cow is fresh and down with twitching muscles and cold ears and depressed (classic signs for milk fever) and someone goes to drench her with a liquid calcium or calcium tube, thinking they can get away with not giving an intravenous (IV) treatment. Not a good idea at all! If a cow is down with milk fever, do *not* drench her; her swallowing muscles are also not working properly, and getting things in the lungs at this point is very easy. And besides, her blood levels are so low (obvious since she cannot rise) that calcium directly into the blood stream is what's needed right then and there. If you don't know how to give an IV bottle of calcium, call the veterinarian, and/or learn how to give one correctly. Then there are milk vein abscesses. As a vet, I actually do use the milk vein for intravenous placement of fluids. And yes, it is all going into the same system as the neck vein (after all it is the same animal)—it is one big circulatory system and it doesn't matter where you insert the needle to deliver the fluids—*if* you do it correctly. Don't ever give a first calf heifer an IV in the milk vein because the vein simply isn't sufficiently developed, so it's very easy to get the fluid next to the vein rather than in the vein. Don't even try it on a mean cow. If you are giving an IV in the milk vein and the cow starts to kick a little, this is her signal to let you know that it is not going in the right place and you ought to stop what you are doing right then and there.

I think you get the idea of what I mean by "loving a cow to death." For most folks it only takes one bad experience with any of the above scenarios to not repeat it. I do want to say that I really appreciate that farmers try to treat their own cows, especially if they do it right. And most of the time things are done right; only once in a while does a problem develop. It's just that over the years, I've seen many of these kinds of problems repeatedly. We need to keep in mind the principle that intervention is not *always* needed. Sometimes an animal just needs a day (one day, not a bunch of days in a row) to see if she'll get better or not. All of us have our down days and animals are no different, especially those in production. Yes, we don't like it that they are not performing at 100 percent all the time, but no one does. I guess as a vet, I prefer using an IV treatment to get a cow stronger more quickly, and I know many of you realize the benefit of knowing how to give an IV versus just giving a pill or drench in the mouth to help a cow. It's been said that a gallon of fluid in the vein is worth ten gallons pumped into the stomach. I agree. Actually a gallon of fluid in the vein *and* ten gallons pumped into the rumen is even better. However, any treatment also needs to be done correctly. Just step back for a minute before glugging some stuff down the cow's throat and think about *why* she might be slow. Learn to address the root cause before applying Band-Aids, especially if they aren't needed.

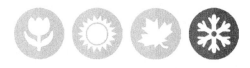

CHAPTER 17

Sprouted Grains

It seems like there's been a lot of talk about sprouted grains over the past few years. Being that I'm not a professionally trained nutrition-ist, I've stayed in the background and simply listened to the chit-chat about it. Probably some of you have done the same. After seeing my first sprouting system and the gusto with which the animals ate the sprouts, I'm an instant supporter! The system I saw was in the south-east Pennsylvania region and set up for a forty-cow dairy. I visited the site with Dr. Silvia Abel-Caines, the ruminant nutritionist for Organic Valley, who has previously done some research with sprouted grains. Some of the information in this chapter comes from a talk she gave at an extremely well-attended meeting sponsored by Organic Valley on November 30, 2012, in Gratz, Pennsylvania. The following are some basics about sprouts.

Perhaps most importantly, feeding spouted grains is feeding fresh, live food. In a sense it is continuing the grazing season in a miniature way through the winter when the cows are inside. In regular grain, there are anti-nutritional factors, such as phytase and tannins, which help the seed protect itself. Just soaking seeds overnight (without actual sprouting) will deactivate the phytase and tannins. I remember seeing a few farmers soaking grain overnight in buckets as many as ten years ago, the idea being that it would be better when fed out. Now I understand why. Regular grain also brings starch into the rumen, which can cause problems like rumen acidosis, whereas sprouted grains provide sugars instead of starch. Starch and sugar are both forms of energy (being sources of carbon), but the sugars are friendlier to the digestion process.

There have been many experiments on how long to grow the sprouted grains. It seems that they should be harvested on day six—easy to remember with the biblical injunction for resting on the seventh day. The biological reality is that the starch reserves of the dry grain are used up by that point. You need soil for any further growth beyond that time. Also, the composition of the plant changes after day six. In general, 285 pounds of dry grain will yield one ton of sprouted grain (with soaked-up water). Thinking purely in dry matter, 1 pound of grain will yield 1.4 pounds of sprouts in six days, *and* it's fresh, green feed.

Let's look at the nutritional profile of sprouts. Crude protein in barley grain is about 13 percent, and about 16 percent when sprouted. Vitamin E, which is critical to proper immune system functioning but universally low in stored feeds, can increase from about 7 milligrams per kilogram in barley grain to 62 milligrams per kilogram when sprouted. Beta-carotene goes from 4.1 milligrams per kilogram in barley grain to 42 milligrams per kilogram when sprouted. Beta-carotene is the starting compound for vitamin A and also has important immune system functions. Biotin, which helps glucose production as well as keratin production for hoof health, increases from 0.16 milligrams per kilogram to 1.15 milligrams per kilogram. Free folic acid, or vitamin B_9, goes from 0.12 milligrams per kilogram to 1.05 milligrams per kilogram. Looking at these numbers, we can see that the actual levels of these nutrients increase ten times within a six-day period, just from sprouting grains.

Being live feed, sprouts also increase enzyme levels, which give better digestion and absorption. As far as protein considerations, soluble protein is converted to bypass protein when grain is sprouted, thus less rumen ammonia to deal with and therefore less milk urea nitro-

Winter manure

Want to try an experiment with some pen manure or gut-ter manure (that's not liquid)? I've read of a low-labor way of making compost by Trauger Groh, a biodynamic farmer in New Hampshire. He does it this way: Make a square pile of winter manure. In May or June, split it into two windrows. Cover with black plastic and make holes on the top so it can breathe. Do not touch it anymore until it is ready for use the following year. Use it the next spring as a fully finished compost. Covering is critical because you don't want it to be too wet. Manure with more than 70 percent moisture cannot build humus. Piles are 6 feet high fresh, made with straw/hay manure, and go down a foot or so as they age. They don't use woodchips or sawdust, but if they did they would only need a little longer composting depending on size of woodchips.

gen (MUNs). Sprouted grains also have increased amino acids, such as glutamine and proline, which are converted to lysine (an amino acid cows cannot make on their own and is normally supplemented). The response of the cows on the farm I visited was obvious in just six weeks' time—with a butterfat level of 4.3 percent and protein at 3.3 per-cent—and this was late November *with Holsteins*.

The action of water alone on regular dry grain is nothing short of miraculous: starch is converted to sugars, proteins are converted to amino acids, and lipids are converted to fatty acids (quality energy). Perhaps most important of all, animals *enjoy* sprouts, as seen by the yearlings ripping at the mats of squares fed to them. With a total mixed ration (TMR), just add the sprouts to the mixer like the farm I visited does.

However, there is one major drawback that comes along with all this goodness: extra labor is necessary—loading the grain into trays and filling them with water, loading the trays onto the shelves, check-ing fodder growth daily, removing the trays from the shelves and emptying them into a container, washing and rinsing trays, and feeding the green feed to the animals. But you can easily make this a part of the daily routine since you feed your animals every day anyway, right? I don't make light of the fact you are feeding your cows everyday anyway as adding a sprouting system does takes prolonged, conscious effort.

You can make your own unit or you can buy them ready-to-go, and apparently they can be financed as a lease (with tax benefits). Commercially ready units go under the names of Almighty Fodder, Fodder Wheel, FodderPro, and FodderTech, among others. The unit I saw on the farm in Pennsylvania was designed by a farmer in Washington State. The farmers feeding sprouts seem to be happy pioneers—their cows, too.

Farmers who wish to try growing sprouted grains must take into consideration the necessity of keeping constant temperature and humidity control to ensure that growth is optimum and molds are inhibited. The temperature should be a steady 70°F (~20°C) and 70 percent humidity. This needs to be monitored continually with gauges mounted on the walls in plain sight. Slope of tray is another important factor to keep in mind for all seeds to germinate properly and not get too waterlogged. Recycling used water for further sprout production is not recommended, but recycling the water for other farm uses is fine. Notably, nothing needs to be added to the water for the sprouts—the starting grain has all the reserves it needs. Simply applying warmth, humidity, and water will start the miracle of life from otherwise dormant, hard-to-digest, dry grain.

Sprouting seeds seems like a great opportunity to get fresh, high-quality feed to your cows year-round. I've always liked eating sprouts myself, and knowing a bit more about them now, I think I'll ramp up my own intake of them!

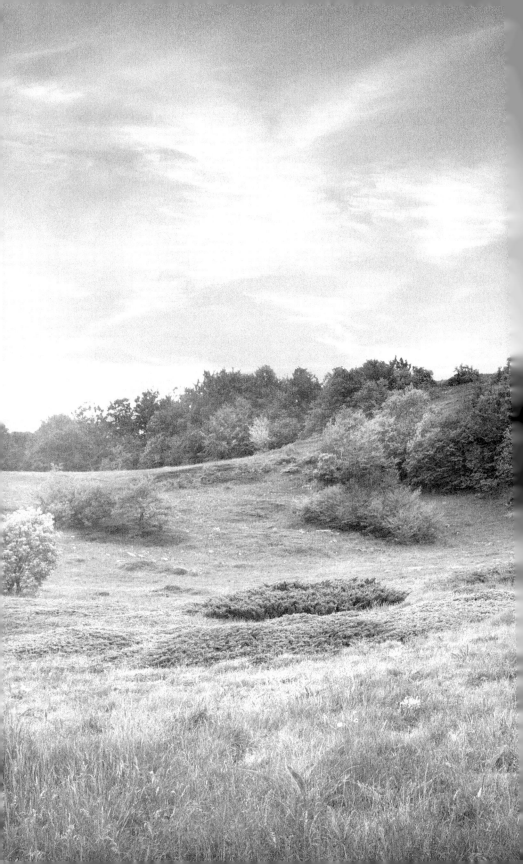

PART V

Any Season

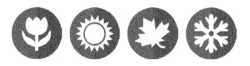

CHAPTER 18

Mastitis

One major health issue I worry about year-round as a vet is mastitis—especially mastitis in dry, near-fresh and fresh cows. With hazy, hot, and humid weather, cases of this devastating disease can strike all of a sudden. Other vets I regularly talk with have confirmed this notion. The effects of humidity on a cow that leaks milk or has a dirty udder spell trouble. Add to this the fact that dry cows are not generally watched as closely until they are mopey and observed not eating right, and quite a disaster is suddenly upon you.

In the summer, dry cows may develop mastitis due to flies on the teat ends or perhaps tramping a teat and not having it noticed by the farmer for a few days. Typically, dry cows tend to get the germs that cause coliform or arcanobacter mastitis. Both these situations can lead to problems not only for the cow but for the calf inside. Mastitis in dry cows usually also causes a fever, probably due to the kind of infection itself and also since she is not getting stripped out like she would during lactation. Springing heifers also can get mastitis with the same results. When the animal is finally tended to, the quarter itself will usually be irreversibly damaged and rock-hard. If it is arcanobacter mastitis, this type of infection usually results in a thick, yellowish, pudding-like secretion that has a very foul odor.

Penicillin can save the life of the cow, as the bug is highly sensitive to it. If prompt attention is given, the cow and developing calf may do okay, but this will not save the quarter once the infection is established. Natural treatments have given positive results for the cow and calf generally as well. My standard treatment is: IV dextrose with 90cc of Get Well (herbal antibacterial mix), 250cc antibodies (Bovi-Sera), 250cc sodium iodide, 500cc vitamin C, and 1cc/100lbs flunixin (Banamine). If this kind of infection is not caught in time, the cow can be generally sick and potentially lose the calf or have a dead calf born. It's impossible to accurately predict whether or not the calf survives to term, is born dead, or is aborted. If the cow aborts, has no udder to speak of, and has penicillin loaded in her, she will make a beef cow later. But not treating arcanobacter mastitis can sometimes lead to gas gangrene mastitis due to the extreme swelling and loss of circulation to the udder and an immediate loss of the animal.

If there is a coliform mastitis (watery, "lemonade-like" secretions) in any cow, the all natural treament of IV dextrose, Get Well, Bovi-Sera, sodium iodide and vitamin C works quite will against coliform mastitis if caught within the first 12 hours of onset. If using antibiotics, use oxytetracycline (LA-200) or ampicillin (both have withholding times), or ceftiofur (Naxcel or Excenel with slight withholding times).

IT IS OF UTMOST IMPORTANCE TO TREAT THESE ANIMALS EARLY to have a functional cow in the future. Coliform bacteria reproduce themselves about every twenty minutes, rapidly increasing their population in the udder.

It is of utmost importance to treat these animals *early* to have a functional cow in the future. Coliform bacteria reproduce themselves about every twenty minutes, rapidly increasing their population in the udder. Slightly off-colored milk can become watery within two to three hours. Treatment also consists of IV fluids, and lots of them. Getting the cow rehydrated or keeping her hydrated is one of the key issues in addressing coliform mastitis. Simply giving a probiotic pill and waiting is *not* a good idea. In addition, anti-inflammatory medication such as aspirin (give five to six pills) or flunixin (Banamine), a cousin to aspirin but a hundred times as powerful, is crucial to helping your cow since flunixin counteracts endotoxins produced by the coliform bacteria: give 1cc per 100 pounds. Also 250cc–500cc of vitamin C to support and stimulate the immune system is very important.

For common mastitis (environmental staphylococcus or environmental streptococcus), when an animal is *not* systemically ill, the botanical/vitamin combination formula of Phyto-Mast can be very helpful. Its active ingredient is essential oil of thyme in a base of licorice, angelica, wintergreen, and vitamins A, D, and E in certified organic olive oil. It is the most studied natural product for food-producing animals in the world. There are four published scientific articles on its safety and efficacy for use against clinical mastitis and drying off cows in peer-reviewed journal articles. However, it is actually a multipurpose product, with farmers using it to cleanse the eye for pinkeye (instead of an antibiotic tube), as a healing antibacterial for those udder sores (clean it up really well first), and also for helping with digestive disturbances in calves. It is manufactured in a facility that is GMP (good manufacturing practices) compliant. At the time of this writing, North Carolina State University is conducting studies to determine the milk and meat withdrawal times for dairy cows. One of the already-published studies described the same in dairy goats.

Just remember—if using nonantibiotic approaches to a quarter with mastitis, by all means keep that quarter out of the bulk tank. This will ensure marketability of your milk as well as helping to achieve quality premium bonuses. Run a CMT (California Mastitis Test) on any cow if you're not sure which quarter is bad.

In fresh cows that leak milk, the heat and humidity along with lying down on wood shavings used for bedding or a lying in a mucky area under a shade tree make for problems. If you have mattresses, do *not* use *any* shavings until the humidity lessens. Simply use lime or

straw/fodder under the cows' back feet upon the mattresses. Straw is fairly inert, if replaced regularly. Sand is totally inert but doesn't work well with gravity flow manure pits. Using straw/fodder will also decrease moisture in the gutter, which will help also reduce fly-growing areas. Also, try adding rock phosphate to the gutter areas to help dry things down. By adding the rock phosphate into the gutter, it will also become biologically activated much sooner than simply applying it to the field from the bag.

Cows bunching up around trees are unfortunately a well-known site to casual observers. Hot coliform mastitis can be the end result of such scenes. It is perhaps better to have no trees in a pasture than a very small amount. Better yet is to plant trees and have them fenced off. One farmer I know has about five acres of dedicated permanent pasture and a few years ago planted willow trees protected by fencing. They have been growing nicely and are all producing a modest amount of shade now. It is nice to see the herd spread themselves out evenly beneath the shade of many trees rather than bunching all together under one tree. When nearly the entire herd of forty cows is standing in the same spot underneath one big tree, I would forecast coliform mastitis to be brewing, especially in the humid and rainy summers on the East Coast. Since some people are entirely opposed to the thought of vaccinating to prevent for illnesses, prevention through wise management of soil, shade, and moisture is paramount. Even with smart management to keep cows in dry areas, if the cows' udders are in contact with wood shavings in their stalls, the potential of contracting coliform mastitis is increased. Add in any leaking water bowls or leaking teats and there is a near certainty that at least one cow will break with a hot mastitis that is actually entirely preventable.

If experiencing hot coliform mastitis, fresh cows need to be treated the same way as dry cows for dehydration and fever. There are many peppermint lotions available, that are very soothing and cooling. Cows seem to like them being applied when they have a hot mastitis. Stripping out all the initial secretions is also important. Using B-vitamins and probiotics to help the appetite and rumen is vital, as is vitamin C as an antioxidant, especially if the rumen is shut down and not creating its own vitamin C.

One area of prevention probably underutilized by many farmers is vaccinating with J-5 to prevent the terrible effects of coliform mastitis. An animal may still get a watery quarter, but there will only be a minimal fever (if any) and the udder won't be rock-hard (only mildly swollen). She will still eat some, the treatment costs will be minimized, and the treatment outcome much improved. I highly recommend vaccinating against coliform if there is a history on the farm of more than one cow per forty affected by it in a year's time. This vaccine also helps prevent calf scours. Just never do any kind of vaccinating on a hot day as the immune system will not process it correctly. Perhaps more importantly, the heat can cause adverse reactions right after vaccinating. Simply wait for a cooler day. Remember, a cow's body temperature peaks about three to four hours after the peak temperature of the day. You can further help your dry cows during the heat by boosting their immune system at dry-off and two weeks before freshening with a shot of vitamin E and selenium (MuSe).

High somatic cell count (SCC) is common and rises and falls with seasonal changes such as heat and humidity or cold and damp conditions. It is always good to get milk cultured to see which germs might be causing the problem. If high SCC is a constant problem (400,000 or higher), consider making a vaccine from the milk of the worst cows. These autogenous vaccines are specific to your herd and I have seen them work exceptionally well where Staph aureus has been a problem. Consult your veterinarian. Alternatively, a homeopathic nosode can be made from the milk and given orally. Also, look at teat ends for any "cheerio" rings that can indicate over-milking (pulling the inside of the teat outwards). They gather dirt easily and can contribute to high SCC.

Cows with high somatic cell counts (SCC) are often experiencing exposure to mastitis, but their immune systems are responding very vigorously—but not so much to cause irregular-looking milk. For high-SCC cows I recommend Biocel-CBT (Agri-Dynamics) given

at the rate of 35cc under the skin for three days in a row, or a dose of ImmunoBoost under the skin one time. Also, massaging in Udder Master, a non-mint udder lotion, can help reduce SCC and mastitis while also softening the udder.

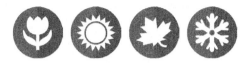

CHAPTER 19

Hardware Disease

A lthough hardware disease occurs throughout the year, I generally see more cases in the winter months, when cows are inside. During this season, people feeding only stored feeds, which during harvest could very well have picked up a variety of foreign objects, whether metal wire, horseshoe nails, screws, small stones, crushed soda cans, or even glass. Of course, cows grazing pastures can also get into trouble along fencelines or if there are areas where things were burned, since there may have been wood with nails or other metallic, unburnable items.

Hardware disease is actually an umbrella term for any foreign object that causes a strong enough traumatic impact to the cow's digestive tract, especially in the area of the reticulum (the first stomach). The worst case as described in veterinary textbooks is called traumatic reticulo-pericarditis, when a sharp object penetrates the wall of the reticulum, piercing the diaphragm as well as the pericardium (sac around the heart). This creates a septic fluid within the pericardium and severely compromises heart function, usually leading to death.

Why is it that cows eat bad things? It's mainly due to the way they take in feed. Watch a cow graze, and you'll see her tongue wraps around a bunch of grass and rips it upward into her mouth. This is because cows don't have upper front teeth to bite with, as horses do. Although sheep and goats don't have upper front teeth either, those two species have nimble and sensitive lips that warn them of sharp objects to avoid. However, hardware disease is not necessarily caused only by sharp metal objects. Similar symptoms of a stopped-up gut can be caused by an accumulation of sand, small pebbles and stones, glass fragments, or any other foreign object large enough to ruin the digestive tract.

The symptoms are typically these: the cow goes abruptly off-feed and milk is reduced to near zero within one to two milkings. A low-grade fever (102.7°F–103.2°F) is usually present, but it can be higher. Only hay is desired, if anything at all. The cow has a humped back, and if you pull up on the skin at the shoulders, the cow will remain humped up because of the pain underneath in the chest. There will be firm/fibrous manure that if squeezed will release droplets of liquid with fibers remaining in hand.

Treatment requires a magnet, which will be swallowed into the reticulum (first stomach) and draw the metal onto itself. Magnets usually stay in the reticulum for life, but sometimes they will pass out. You can check to see if a cow has a magnet already by crouching in front of her brisket with a compass and seeing if the needle points directly toward the brisket. (Make sure the cow is not standing directly north of you!) By the way, one magnet alone has more "pull" than two or more together. If you don't believe me, place one magnet on a metal post and pull it away and then try it with two or more magnets together. The group of magnets will be easier to pull off than the single one.

As would be expected, a rusty or dirty piece of metal piercing through internal organs can cause an infection. If the metal pierces through to the heart area, the prognosis is very poor, especially if heart function is so compromised that the milk veins become engorged and edema of the brisket and under the jaw (bottle jaw) occurs. The jugular veins will look very full, and you'll see "waves" of pulsing blood going upward with each heartbeat. If the metal pierces the lungs instead, some pulmonary abscesses will probably develop. If the metal pierces not the chest cavity but the abdominal cavity, there will be an initial infection (peritonitis), then scarring of the reticulum to its adjacent organs—the liver, rumen, or abomasum.

Giving a strong magnet one time and a strong antibacterial tincture two to three times a day for four to five days can work well. Farmers are quick to give magnets, which is good to stop the problem early. In general, if the cow was milking at peak, she could be expected to get back to about 80 percent of where she was in about two weeks' time. Cows affected later in lactation may not come back well and will dry off early. And periodic bloating is a possibility after hardware since the vagus nerve, which stimulates the rumen to function, can be damaged.

THE IDEA OF GIVING all cows a magnet at first breeding as a heifer or at first freshening is a good one, but few farmers do it.

The traditional surgery for extracting the offending piece of metal is rarely done in the barn these days, as it is very involved. However, I did have a surprise once while doing a twisted stomach surgery. I was doing my normal sweep of the internal area before sewing the stomach down, and, lo and behold, I discovered a nail poking out of the reticulum and pulled it out. It was a horseshoe nail, very rusty at that. It was only the second time that I've actually extracted a nail from a cow, and it was only a chance finding while correcting a twist. Another practitioner I talked with said that he once pulled a nail out of the pylorus (outlet of the fourth stomach) after sewing the stomach down.

The idea of giving all cows a magnet at first breeding as a heifer or at first freshening is a good one, but few farmers do it. One magnet costs between $2–$4; multiplied by fifty cows, the practice will cost you $100–$200 in prevention, and that is cheap compared to losing a cow to hardware. If the cause of the "hardware" disease is an accumulation of irritating small stones, glass, or nonmagnetic metal (aluminum

soda cans, usually crumpled and sharp), a magnet will unfortunately not help. Nonetheless, for less than $5 per cow, giving a magnet is well worth the money.

By the way, there are other conditions that can look like hardware. Cancer certainly can put a cow off-feed, but usually only moderately, with small recoveries over a few to many weeks. You can usually detect enlarged lymph nodes (either internally or externally), and the cow will be slow to rise and may grind her teeth. A cow with a stomach ulcer is another possibility. A humpback on a fresh, young cow milking really well and grinding her teeth and being pushed hard with lots of grain would be such a suspect. If it's a bleeding ulcer, the manure will be black and tar-like, accompanied by a fever. A kidney infection can give a humpback, fever, and put a cow off-feed. This problem can be initiated by a bad uterus after calving, with the septic fluid making its way in reverse through the bladder and back to the kidneys. An odd condition, mesenteric torsion (early), can display symptoms similar to hardware, but within a day they will kick at the belly with complete blockage of the intestines and no manure at all. Spoiled feed will put a cow off-feed until she blasts out with profuse, watery scours a day or two later, and then she will start eating again. Unexplained sudden death may be attributed to hardware (or internal bleeding).

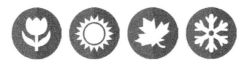

CHAPTER 20

Rabies

Usually with warm weather, but really anytime, many wild creatures are moving about and living out their lives in the nearby woods. Unfortunately, along with woodland animal activity and interaction comes the increased possibility of rabies transmission. Rabies is a viral infection that can take anywhere from twenty days to six months to incubate in the bitten victim. Once it shows itself clinically, there is no way to reverse the course of the disease. The end result is always death. The common signs are episodes of odd behavior (aggressive or depressed), overly friendly activity for a wild animal, odd vocal sounds, reluctance or inability to drink water, salivating, drooling, and/or foaming at the mouth. Once the signs are observable, the animal will die in about five to ten days. There is no recovery with rabies. So if an animal is displaying these symptoms, but then improves, it isn't rabies.

The usual carriers are raccoons, foxes, skunks, and bats. As a licensed veterinarian I get a complete listing of all tested rabies positive cases in Pennsylvania counties every month. The entire listing usually includes a couple dogs, cats, a cow or two, a horse, a mule, a few opossums, and

IF A VACCINATED DOG OR CAT gets into a fight with a raccoon or skunk (or whatever wild animal) that wanders into the barn, barnyard, or farmstead, we immediately revaccinate your pet. You need to do it quickly—not a week later when you get around to doing it.

maybe a groundhog—in addition to scores of raccoons and skunks. Bats are hard to catch to test. If bitten by a bat, assume it is rabid and seek medical attention. Any nocturnal animal (animal that is usually active at night) that is seen active and/or acting oddly in the daytime should be considered as a possibly infected animal. One time, at noon when I was sitting by the Octorara Creek, a bat was flying overhead. Not good. Another time during the day I saw a raccoon doing back flips in a recently harvested corn field. A few summers ago, at midday, a raccoon came within ten feet of my front porch, making really weird noises and odd backwards jumps right near my cat, which was about three feet away from it. I quickly took a metal bucket and threw it at the coon and off it went. But I was on high alert the rest of the day and carried a baseball bat around with me in the yard. Never did see that coon again, but I told the neighbors to stay on alert.

Pennsylvania state law requires that all dogs and domestic cats be vaccinated against rabies. However, the Pennsylvania Farm Bureau successfully lobbied to keep barn cats exempt since it would be too costly for farmers to spend the time and labor to gather them up to get vaccinated. And yet as we all know, it is barn cats most likely to come up against a wild animal trespassing in the barn. The recommended vaccination for *all* dogs is for their first shot no younger than three months of age, then a booster a year later, then every three years thereafter. I carry vaccines for dogs and cats (it's the only small animal vaccine that I carry) and will gladly vaccinate farm dogs and other animals. State law mandates that a licensed veterinarian admin-

ister the vaccine for the animal to be considered officially vaccinated.
However, licensed kennel owners can get permission to vaccinate
their own dogs if they have been shown how to properly do it by their
veterinarian. There is no state law requiring a veterinarian to adminis-
ter the vaccine to farm production animals like cows and horses. You
can vaccinate your own cows and horses, if you feel inclined. Hardly
any farmers do this locally, but in other states they do.*

If a *vaccinated* dog or cat gets into a fight with a raccoon or skunk
(or whatever wild animal) that wanders into the barn, barnyard, or
farmstead, we immediately revaccinate your pet. You need to do it
quickly—not a week later when you get around to doing it. Usually
people get frightened, and rightfully so, when they see odd behavior
by a wild animal in the yard. Boosting the initial vaccine will send
the antibodies into high gear and protect your pet. Those antibodies
were created from the first vaccination. If, however, your pet was not
vaccinated, it must stay in strict quarantine for six months so it can be
determined whether your pet will come down with the virus or not.
Unfortunately, most farmers will not do a strict quarantine and the
unfortunate animal is put to sleep. A previous vaccination would have
prevented that.

If a human was exposed to an animal that tested rabies positive, the
state public health department will come to your farm and figure out
who needs to get the post-exposure series of shots. These will save the
life of the person who has accidentally gotten any bit saliva or blood
of the rabid animal into any nicks or cuts on the skin. If I am involved,
as I was when putting a yearling heifer down a few years ago that
tested positive for rabies, I also get a booster shot (the same as would a
properly vaccinated dog) since I am already vaccinated due to my line
of work. (And no, I don't have any official vaccination paper or rabies
tag for myself!)

Remember that vaccinating for rabies is state law. A rabies vaccination paper isn't the same as a county dog license. They are separate but

---

* For each state's rules on rabies vaccination, see https://www.avma.org/Advo-
cacy/StateAndLocal/Pages/rabies-vaccination.aspx.

both are required by law, otherwise you could face some pretty stiff fines by the dog officer. The dog tags that I dispense after vaccinating a dog have my clinic name and phone number on it so that if your dog wanders off, the person who finds it can call me and I can look up the record and say who it belongs to. This has helped reunite dog and owner half a dozen times in the last year. The more important piece of evidence to have is the piece of paper that I fill out that proves the dog was officially vaccinated against rabies. This is critical in case your dog bites someone.

As is clear, the rabies vaccine is important, both immunologically as well as legally. But like any vaccine, there can potentially be side-effects if vaccinated too frequently. While too frequent vaccination is not a likely case with rabies vaccination (as it could be with the 10-way vaccines farmers use against respiratory and reproductive problems), I have heard from some veterinarians that an occassional horse had developed angry behavior and a changed character when vaccinated repeatedly against rabies. This should not stop a person from using the rabies vaccine, however. Instead, after giving the vaccine, give the homeopathic nosode Lyssin orally. It is made from rabies virus but potentized like any other homeopathic product to the point where there is no starting material remaining (once higher than a 12C or 24X). Use the Lyssin 200C one time after a rabies vaccine injection to blunt negative side effects from developing. The idea of following a vaccination with a homeopathic nosode to blunt side effects can be done for any condition actually.

Rabies is entirely preventable by vaccination. It is one of the few vaccines that I urge to be used, not only because it can prevent such a dreaded disease but because it is also state law.

Conclusion
Happy New Year

To ring in the New Year and close out the old, let's begin by realizing how lucky we are to be involved with the organic industry. Consider this: between 2000 and 2010, there was an average of 20 percent per year growth in organics. And during an absolutely terrible year for conventional dairy, and the economy in general (2009), organics still showed growth, even if only by 1 percent. Since then, the organic sector, and especially demand for organic milk has regained a robust growth rate. I'm not saying that we should look backward—not at all. But sometimes when everything seems to have gone wrong in so many places in the world, we should for a moment look at how far we've come as organic farmers, organic agricultural professionals, and organic advocates.

Think back to when you were transitioning (and for some of you that may have been pretty recently)—weren't you really worried about what would happen to your crops when you stopped using herbicides, insecticides, and fungicides? And now, whether a year or two into being certified or already ten to fifteen years certified, think about all the chemical sprays that you're *not* using. Granted the expense for them is gone, but even better so are the dangers to your health when mixing and applying them. Isn't it pretty amazing that you *can* farm without all those chemicals that people previously told you that you simply had to use to get crops in? Your horses, cows, and other farm animals are healthier for your choice to go organic as well—both by not being in contact with the sprays and by eating feeds that were not sprayed either.

And what about your soil? Once the winter freeze gives up its grip when spring hits, go and dig a few holes when your soil is warmed up. Pick up a clod of topsoil and look at it closely. Look for the channels that roots and small insects have left behind. These channels are the means by which water can percolate down through your soil instead of ponding on the surface. How many earthworms do you see? Ideally there should be about twenty-five per cubic foot. Organic soils, simply by not being sprayed with toxic compounds to kill things, will of course contain more biological life. Fertilizers like ammonium nitrate and anhydrous ammonia (conventional fertilizer) may give a quick jump start to plants, but they are deadly to soil organisms. Additionally you will create a hard surface, which will hinder water penetration. Now that you're organic, I'll bet you think about the life of your soil a lot more than when you were conventional. And why not? Live soil is where it all starts—organic philosophy promotes this constantly.

As the saying goes, healthy soils grow vigorous crops, which yield nutritious feed for animals and people. Yet it's also true that poorly managed soils grow weak crops, which yield questionable food for animals and people. In poorly aerated soils, molds have a much easier time establishing themselves. I've always been a fan of disking in cover crops and manure and using a deep ripping implement like a chisel or yeoman plow to create shafts in the soil to allow air, water, and roots to penetrate down.

Now let's think about the animals in the barn. Weren't you *really* worried about health problems prior to starting organic management of your cows? It is still a common concern for those thinking about transitioning. But how many animals do you cull involuntarily in a year nowadays? I would guess that it is fewer than when farming conventionally and using conventional treatments. While you are now probably much more aware of the occasional problem that pops up when farming organically, from direct experience with organic herds I will say that there are *dramatically fewer* problems overall. In general, I've found that at about two years after certification, things *really* begin to smooth out for the long term. While your herd may not be peaking as high (rolling herd average), I would also guess that you are retaining more when it comes to the bottom line without having to always add cows. Hey, at the least, your milk check doesn't swing like in the conventional setting. That alone is a lot less stress for you—and less stress will keep you, your family, and your farm animals healthier in the long run.

How about all the conventional treatments that you previously used for reproduction—think of all the shots to help cows get bred back. Were you using new needles on every cow—or at least sanitizing them each and every time? If not, each shot potentially passed disease onto the next cow. Now think about all those shots with the synchronization programs. Do you really miss them? While organic management demands more intense labor on your part (especially for fresh cows that might not have cleaned), you probably have come to realize that good, old visual inspection of your cows will tell you which cows are in heat or near heat. Probably the number one thing for cows to show heat and get bred back, organic or conventional, is proper body condition (rather than using shots).

And what about mastitis? Granted, by the very nature of milking cows, every dairy farm will have ups and downs with milk quality problems. And yes, you do need to do something if things are troublesome just to keep your milk processor happy. But how about all those antibiotic dry cow tubes you used previously. Do you really miss them? And yes, there will be an occasional organic cow at dry off that has real problems—but on average, I will guess that they don't. A study done here in Lancaster County, Pennsylvania in 2007 showed no significant differences between conventional and organic in milk quality for cows one to forty days in milk. Think for a moment about what that means: it is likely that *no* dry-off antibiotics, in general, are needed since both conventional and organic cows begin lactation with the same good milk quality.

Organic definitely requires better attention to detail to keep your crops and animals healthy. But in organics you are free from that ball-and-chain reliance on herbicides, fungicides, insecticides, synchronizing hormonal shots, and the routine use of antibiotics that are so prevalent in agriculture. By not relying on chemicals and drugs, you are free to rely more on your own vision, intellect, and fortitude to steer your farm. By combining my previous college and now updated knowledge of soil and crop science (thanks to Midwestern Bio-Ag and the Rodale Institute) with my direct, in-the-barn veterinary animal health expertise, it's fairly easy for me to see how all the pieces of "the puzzle" fit together. Does your nutritionist link what you feed to how it was grown? It does all begin with smart management of your soil, coaxing its natural existing fertility by improving its structure (vitally important) and enhancing the living biology within it to unleash its potential to grow vibrant and diverse crops. Add nutrients only if short in them! Why spend for things that could end up in our oceans? Many soils already have more than enough phosphorus and potassium. And if the soils are truly alive and vigorous, you might even be able to do without a nitrogen application occasionally. But you have to "earn the right" (as Gary Zimmer likes to say), mainly by enlivening your farm's soils. So why add only NPK every year? After all, it is usually the calcium, sulfur, boron, and other micronutrients that really what makes the difference when it comes to quality feed. Feeding home-grown, nutrient-dense (good mineral levels) crops with a forage-to-grain ration of 60:40 or 65:35 is a fundamental building block to nourishing healthy cows able to overcome the common stresses that can occur. These last points are hallmarks of organic agriculture. Contrast this to how things were done on your farm before going organic. I'll bet that you are actually pretty content, paid fairly, and glad to know that you produce food for society while keeping the land and animals healthy and clean. Let's keep growing organically to create a cleaner world that our children are happy to inherit.

Sources of Products

Phyto-Mast™, Udder Master, Get Well, Eat Well, Liv Well, Heat Seek, Ferro, Homeopathic remedies
CowMaster, LLC
Hubert Karreman, VMD
555 Red Hill Road
Narvon, Pennsylvania 17555
Phone: 717-405-8137 for Dr. Karreman; 1-844-209-COWS (2697) for CowMaster, LLC products
E-mail: penndutch@earthlink.net
Website: www.hubertkarreman.com

Biocel-CBT, Ketonic, Phyto-Biotic, Vermi-Tox, Neema-Tox, Ecto-Phyte, Dyna-min, Dyna-vites, HemoCel 100, Graziers Essentials, Native Lick, Aqua Nox, Flies-Be-Gone, Winter-Mune
Agri-Dynamics
P.O. Box 267
6574 South Delaware Drive
Martins Creek, Pennsylvania 18063
Phone: 610-250-9280 or 877-393-4484
E-mail: info@agri-dynamics.com
Website: www.agri-dynamics.com

ImmunoBoost™: NovaVive USA Inc., Athens, Georgia. This product is available from veterinarians and is technically over-the counter.

Maxi/Guard™ pinkeye bacterin and Autogenous vaccines (custom made from your herd):
Addison Biological Laboratory, Inc.
507 North Cleveland Avenue
Fayette, Missouri 65248
Phone: 660-248-2215 or 800-331-2530
Fax: 660/ 248-2554
E-mail: info@addisonlabs.com

Bovi-Sera
This product is available from veterinarians and is technically over-the counter.
Colorado Serum Company
P.O. Box 16428
4950 York Street
Denver, Colorado 80216-0428
Phone: 800-525-2065
Fax: 303-295-1923
E-mail: colorado-serum@colorado-serum.com

Any good farm supply store or www.enasco.com: Stomach pump, stethoscope, magnets, IV line, electric prod, urine ketone strips, calving chains, calf tube feeder, butane powered dehorner (Portosol), infusion pipettes, teat dilators, pill gun, syringes, needles. Injectable vitamin A, D & E; B-complex; vitamin B_{12} (low potency); vaccines, calcium gel tubes; pink laxative pills, mineral oil (as a lubricant); alcohol and alcohol prep pads; 23% calcium, dextrose, hypertonic saline; poloxalene (for pasture bloat); activated charcoal.

Allowed for organic Rx & other products from your local veterinarian: flunixin (Banamine), butorphanol (Torbugesic/Dolorex), xylazine (Rompun/Anased), tolazoline (Tolazine); MuSe, Bovi-Sera, Vaccines, povidone-iodine (Betadine), injectable sodium iodide, iodine antiseptic pills (I.O.Dine pills), vitamin B_{12} (high potency), vitamin C, vitamin K, epinephrine, CMPK, Cal-Phos #2, Lactated ringers solution, sodium iodide, poloxalene (Therabloat). Also: Stomach pump, stethoscope, magnets, IV line, electric prod, urine ketone strips, calving chains, calf tube feeder, butane powered dehorner (Portasol), infusion pipettes, teat dilators, pill gun, syringes, needles Injectable Vitamin A, D & E; vitamin B-complex; calcium gel tubes; pink laxative pills, mineral oil (as a lubricant); alcohol and alcohol prep pads; 23% calcium, dextrose, hypertonic saline; activated charcoal

Don't hesitate to contact your local vet if you are worried or concerned about the health and well-being of your animals. Your local vet knows your herd and animals and can examine them to determine the likely and/or exact problem – and can suggest or provide appropriate treatment on the spot. There is nothing better than a hands-on physical exam to determine the best course of action.

Dr. Karreman is in clinical practice in the Lancaster, PA area and is happy to help you and/or your local veterinarian with questions via email or phone – see the first listing above for contact information.

Index

low-levels of exposure to, 94–95
prevention and treatment of, 95–97
signs and symptoms of, 94–95
tube feeding of, 20–21, 24, 25
vaccination of, 20
Calving and freshening, 3–18. *See also* Milk
    fever; Placenta
area for, 8–9
breech births, 11
cow's body condition during, 4
death of calf, 10–11, 12–13, 202
delivery procedure, 9–13
as displaced abomasum cause, 145–146
duration of, 9
in first-calf heifers, 10, 12
head snare/loop use in, 10–11
during hot weather, 149
ketosis during, 31
normal, 4
on pasture, 190
presentation of calf during, 10–12
problems during, 10–13
signs of onset of, 7, 9
teat dipping prior to, 6, 7
timing of, 24
twin births, 12, 145, 190
unnecessary interventions in, 191–192
uterine contractions during, 189–190, 191
uterine injury during, 11
vaccinations prior to, 4–5, 188–189
Camomile, 71
Canada thistle, 58
Cancer, distinguished from hardware
    disease, 210
Carbohydrates, 117–118
Carbon, 195
Carbon-to-nitrogen ratio, 29, 45
Carb Veg, 76, 77
Cardamon, 71
Carrots, 71
Cats, rabies vaccination of, 212, 213
Caulophyllum, 189–190
Ceftiofur, 176, 202
Celandine, 32–33
Celery, 71
Certification, organic
antibiotic therapy and, 176, 181
National Organic Program (NOP)
    regulations for, 42, 181
Chamomile, 71
Chasteberry, 71
Chenopodium ambrosioides (lambsquarters), 54
nutrient content of, 60
Chickens, use in pasture parasite control,
    49, 96, 126

Chicory, 62, 63
nutrient content of, 60
Chico State University, 100
Chinese chestnut leaves, nutrient content, 61
Choline, 33
Clay, 56–57
Cleavers, nutrient content of, 60
Clostridium Type A, 143
Clover
as bloat cause, 75–76
effect of frost on, 158
as energy source, 34
grazing height of, 34, 54, 126–127
CMPK (calcium, magnesium, phosphorus,
    potassium), 81–82
Cobalt deficiency, 155
Coccidia, 26–27, 91, 93, 173–174
Coccidiostats, 26
Cocklebur, 58
Colchium, 77
Colic, 76, 147–148
Coliform vaccination, 4–5, 186, 189, 205
Colocynthis, 76, 77
Colostrum, 4–5, 20–21
antibodies in, 21, 27, 188
calves' intake of, 191
calves' requirements for, 188
sources of, 23
tube feeding of, 20–21
Colostrum-whey products, 185–186
Comfrey, 60
Component feeding, anionic salts content
    in, 5–6
Compost, 196
Conjugated linoleic acids (CLAs), 40–41
Copper deficiency, 154
Copper sulfate baths, 87
Corn feeding, of grazing cows, 46
Corn silage, 34–35, 45–46
combined with grain feeds, 47
comparison with sorghum-sudan grass, 52
as fiber and energy source, 80
Corn smut *(Ustilago maydis)*, 141
Corpus luteum, 0, 153
Cough. *See also* Pneumonia
in calves, 159–160, 165, 172
treatment for, 168
CowMaster, 177
Cows. *See also* Heifers
gestation period of, 3
herb/tincture dosages for, 69–70
teeth (dentition) of, 208
Cryptosporidia, 26
Cud chewing, 83–84, 85
in calves, 122

Fat, as energy source, 30, 32
Fatty acids, 40–41, 82–83
Feed
    cost of, 39
    cows' daily intake of, 39
    dry cows' intake of, 187–188
    moldy, 141–142, 146
    spoiled, 210
Feed changes
    cows' adjustment to, 140–141
    feeding hay during, 143–144, 145
    problems caused by, 139–148
Feeding, during winter, 139–148
Feeds and Feeding (Morrison), 46
Fenbendazole, 26–27, 99, 172
Fennel, 70
Ferro, 26, 73, 99
Fertilizers, 216, 218
Fertrell's dewormer mix, 99
Fescue, 53
Fever
    as contraindication to injectable
        vaccines, 167
    enzootic calf pneumonia-related, 170
    hardware disease-related, 208
    heat stroke-related, 113–114
    during lactation, 145
    mastitis-related, 188, 201, 205
    pneumonia-related, 175, 177, 178, 181
    scours-related, 142
    uterine infection-related, 145
Fiber, 34, 80
    cows' need for, 144
    cud chewing of, 83–84
    inadequate intake of, 87
First Defense, 5, 21, 23
Fish, Pierre, 69–70
Flash grazing, 79
Flies, 91, 97–99
    control of, 98–99, 100–101, 106–107, 126
    on dehorned/debudded sites, 122
    as mastitis cause, 201
    as pinkeye cause, 103–105, 106–107
    types of, 98
Florfenicol, 176
Fluid therapy. *See* Intravenous (IV)
        fluid therapy
Flunixin (Banamine), 177, 202, 203
Fly repellents, 106
Fly sprays, 98–99, 101, 106
FodderPro, 197
FodderTech, 197
Fodder Wheel, 197
Folic acid, free, 195
Foot rot, 87

Forage-to-grain ration, 218
Foraging behavior, of cows, 56
Foreign objects, in digestive tracts.
        See Hardware disease
Fougère, Barbara, 70–71
Fresh air, role in health maintenance, 132,
        133, 135, 137, 157, 168
Fresh cows. *See also* Calving and freshening
    mastitis in, 201–202
    pinkeye in, 104–105
Freshening. *See* Calving and freshening
Fritz, Tim, 39
Frost
    effect on forage plants, 75
    grazing after, 158
Frostbite, 159

Gaia Herbs, 65
Garlic, 71, 99–100, 177, 178
Gentian, 147
Gestation periods, of livestock, 3
Get Well, 70, 177, 178–179, 202
Giardia, 26, 71
Ginger/ginger root, 70, 71, 99–100, 147
Gingko, 71
Ginseng, 71, 178
Glutamine, 196
Glycerin, 32, 66
Glycerites, 67, 68–69
Goats
    FAMACHA test of, 95
    gestation period of, 3
    herbal medicine dosages for, 70
    stomach worms in, 92
    teeth (dentition) of, 208
Goldenseal, 70, 71, 178
Gonadorelin-releasing hormone, 16, 151
Grain
    as energy source, 84
    sprouted, 194–197
    undigested, 34
Grain feeding
    combined with fiber, 84–85
    combined with forage/fiber, 139–140
    effect on milk production, 139–140
    of grazing cows, 46–48
    during hot weather, 117–118
    as rumen acidosis cause, 34, 44, 46, 47, 84–85
Grain-free grass-fed management
        systems, 47–48
Grape vinegar, 67
Grasses, grazing height of, 126–127
Grass tetany, 80–82
Grazing
    in autumn and winter, 158

Housing. *See also* Barns; Hutches, for calves;
Pens, for calves
air quality/ventilation in, 160
cinder block, 171–172
drafts in, 158, 160
for pneumonia prevention, 172–174
respiratory disease transmission in, 160
Humidity
as mastitis risk factor, 201, 203
for sprouted grain growth, 197
Humus, 196
Hutches, for calves, 19, 20
effect on respiratory health, 168, 173
in hot weather, 119
individual *versus* multi-calf, 173–174
parasite control in, 26
during winter, 158
Hydration, in heat stress, 115
Hypericum, 108
Hyper-immune plasma, 108
Hypocalcemia. *See* Calcium, deficiency/
low-levels of

IBR, 133
Immune system, 4, 165–181
during drying-off period, 182–183, 186
effect of antibiotics on, 140
effect of nutrition on, 166
effect of parasites on, 94, 96, 123–124
effect of selenium deficiency on, 154
effect of vaccination on, 132, 134
energy intake and, 94
in ketosis, 166
in pinkeye, 104
in pneumonia, 167–168
in respiratory disease, 166–167
Immune system stimulants, 25, 166, 177,
178, 186, 189, 205–206
Immunity, in "open" *versus* "closed" herds,
135–136
ImmunoBoost, 25, 166, 178, 186, 189,
205–206
Infections
hardware disease-related, 208
uterine, 145
calving-related, 13, 16–17
displaced abomasum and, 147
effect on breeding, 151
InForce 3, 20, 160, 168
Interferon, 166, 178
Intravenous (IV) fluid therapy, 193
for diarrhea, 145
for heat stroke, 115
for mastitis, 203
for milk fever, 192

for scours, 25
Iodine, 105
as fly repellent, 106
for navel infection prevention, 8–9
Iron, 26, 99
Ivermectin, 26–27, 95–96, 99, 100, 172

J-5, 4–5, 27, 189
Jersey cows, calcium requirements of, 55–56
Jimsonweed, 59
Johne's disease, 20
as diarrhea cause, 155
prevention of, 49
transmission of, 22, 93

Kelp, 56–57, 105, 106–107
Keratin, 195
Ketones, 30–31
Ketosis, 29–35
causes of, 142–143
clinical, 30–32
definition of, 30
in dry cows, 187–188
immune system in, 166
nervous, 30
prevention of, 33–35, 169
primary, 30
secondary, 30
signs of, 143
subclinical, 30, 31, 35
treatment for, 31–33
Kidney infections, 210

Lachesis, 16
Lachesis muta, 152
Lactated ringers solution, 115, 145
Lactation
diet during, 6
displaced abomasum during, 145–146
in first-calf heifers, 21–22
inadequate energy intake during.
See Ketosis
net energy for (NE$_L$), 140
somatic cell counts during, 189
staphylococcal infections during, 186–187
uterine infection treatment during, 17
Lactic acid, 82
Lactobacillus, 141
Lamb's quarters *(Chenopodium ambrosioides),* 54
nutrient content of, 60
Lameness, 86
Laminitis, 154
Legumes
as bloat cause, 59, 75–76
nonbloating, 63

Lemonbalm, 71
Lepto hardjo-bovis, 135
Leptospirosis, 134, 152–153, 155
Lespedeza, 63
Lice, 91
Licorice, 70, 71, 147, 203
Lidocaine, 109, 122–123
Lime
    field, as fly repellent, 98, 107
    hydrated, for hoof health, 87
Liver tonics, 32–33
Longevity, in cows, 118
Lungs
    consolidation of, 174, 180, 181, 192
    metal object-related injuries to, 208–209
Lutalyse (dinoprost), 16, 153
Lymphocytes, 167
Lysine, 196

Macrophages, 166–167
Magnesium, 6, 56–57
    deficiency of, 80–82
    as grass tetany treatment, 81
Magnesium oxide, 81
Magnesium sulfate, 81
Magnets, as hardware disease treatment,
    208, 209–210
Manganese, deficiency of, 155
Mange, 91
Mannheimia hemolytica, 171
Manure
    from cows with stomach ulcers, 210
    disking into soil, 216
    as fly attractant, 97
    in hardware disease, 208
    from healthy cows, 83
    from ketotic cows, 30–31, 143
    "pasture," 80, 83, 84
    relationship to nutrient absorption, 45
    winter, as compost, 196
Manure patties, parasites in, 20, 26, 93, 96
    control of, 38, 49, 100, 102, 126
Manure pits, 170
    gravity flow, 204
Massey University, New Zealand, 62, 63
Mastitis, 6, 201–206
    antibiotic treatment for, 202
    coliform, 4–5
        arcanobacter, 201–202
        distinguished from heat stroke, 114
        in dry cows, 201
        with heat stroke, 114
        prevention of, 203–204
        treatment for, 179, 202–203, 204–205
        vaccination against, 186, 189, 205

    in dry cows, 188, 201
    during dry-off period, 185–187
    environmental, 190, 203
    in fresh cows, 201
    gas gangrene, 188, 202
    natural treatments for, 186–187, 202–203
    in organic *versus* conventional dairy herds,
        217–218
    prevention of, 203–204
    Staphylococcus aureus-related, 136
    vaccination against, 205
Mattresses, 203–204
MaxGuard, 105–106
Mesenteric torsion, 210
Methaplex, 33
Micotil, 176
Micronutrients, 218
    deficiencies in, effect on breeding, 154–155
Midwestern Bio-Ag, 218
Milk
    fat content. *See also* Butterfat
        effect of grazing on, 40–41
    organic, demand for, 215
Milk fever
    as contraindication to drenching, 192
    distinguished from heat stroke, 114
    with grass tetany, 81
    with heat stroke, 114, 115
    in older cows, 7
    prevention of, 5–6, 169, 190
    signs of, 17
    subclinical, 190
    treatment for, 192
Milking, during drying-off period, 184
Milking cows, outdoor *versus* barn housing
    for, 158–159
"Milking the fat off the back," 29–30
Milk production
    21,000 pounds per year, 39
    decrease in, 123
    during drying-off period, 184, 185
    effect of grain feeding on, 139–140
    grain:milk ratio and, 47
    in hardware disease, 208
    during hot weather, 113
    on organic farms, 39
Milk quality. *See also* Somatic cell counts
    (SCCs)
    at dry off, 186
    organic compared with conventional, 218
    in zinc deficiency, 154
Milk thistle, 32–33
Milk urea nitrogen (MUN), 44–45, 80,
    195–196
Milk vein, abscesses of, 192

About the Author

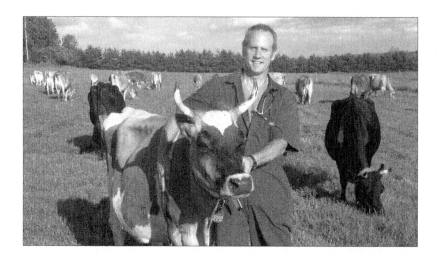

D r. Hubert Karreman is a veterinarian and independent educator of organic veterinary medicine based in Lancaster, Pennsylvania. An active member in many organizations that promote the health and welfare of animals, he is an internationally recognized expert in the non-antibiotic treatment of infectious disease and non-hormonal treatment of infertility. Dr. Karreman graduated in 1995 from the University of Pennsylvania School of Veterinary Medicine. He completed a five-year term on the USDA National Organic Standards Board (2005–2010), serving three years as Chair of the NOSB Livestock Committee. In 1999-2000 Dr. Karreman was on the AVMA Taskforce for Complementary and Alternative Veterinary Medicine (CAVM), which wrote the current AVMA Guidelines on CAVM. Dr. Karreman works with farmers, students, and researchers all over the world to promote ecologically based methods of dairy farming and create a better world for farm animals.

Also by the author

The Barn Guide to Treating Dairy Cows Naturally

HUBERT J. KARREMAN, V.M.D.

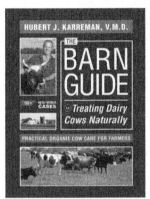

A hands-on guide designed for quick and easy use. Presents a thorough examination of animals in the barn, lists symptoms with many pictures, and shares possible conclusions and treatments that Dr. Karreman has found to work consistently during his years of working with organic cows. Introduces the fundamentals of organic and holistic thinking about livestock. The companion guide to *Treating Dairy Cow Naturally*, this book includes a physical exam section, with nearly 100 case studies organized by symptom and valuable field-tested natural treatments. Color photographs throughout book.

ISBN 978-1-60173-023-7
Softcover • 191 pages • $40.00

Treating Dairy Cows Naturally

HUBERT J. KARREMAN, V.M.D.

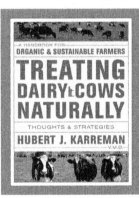

Dr. Karreman describes how cows can be treated for a wide variety of problems with plant-derived and biological medicines. Drawing upon veterinary treatments from before synthetic pharmaceuticals, and tempering them with modern knowledge and clinical experience, this encyclopedic work bridges the world of natural treatments with life in the barn in a rational and easy-to-understand way. In describing treatments for common dairy cow diseases, he covers practical aspects of biologics, botanical medicines, homeopathic remedies, acupuncture and conventional medicine.

ISBN 978-1-60173-000-8
Hardcover • 412 pages • $40.00

**Available from the publisher at www.acresusa.com
and booksellers everywhere.**

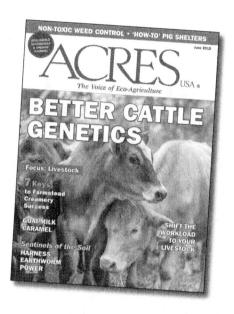

CPSIA information can be obtained at www.ICGtesting.com
Printed in the USA
BVOW06s1345031215

429071BV00002B/11/P